BEYOND THE EMPTINESS

How I Found Fullness
Outside of Food

ROUBA CHALABI

BALBOA.PRESS

A DIVISION OF HAY HOUSE

Balboa Press books may be ordered through booksellers or by contacting:

Balboa Press
A Division of Hay House
1663 Liberty Drive
Bloomington, IN 47403
www.balboapress.com
1 (877) 407-4847

Because of the dynamic nature of the Internet, any web addresses or links contained in this book may have changed since publication and may no longer be valid. The views expressed in this work are solely those of the author and do not necessarily reflect the views of the publisher, and the publisher hereby disclaims any responsibility for them.

The author of this book does not dispense medical advice or prescribe the use of any technique as a form of treatment for physical, emotional, or medical problems without the advice of a physician, either directly or indirectly. The intent of the author is only to offer information of a general nature to help you in your quest for emotional and spiritual well-being. In the event you use any of the information in this book for yourself, which is your constitutional right, the author and the publisher assume no responsibility for your actions.

Any people depicted in stock imagery provided by Getty Images are models, and such images are being used for illustrative purposes only.
Certain stock imagery © Getty Images.

Print information available on the last page.

ISBN: 978-1-9822-5017-1 (sc)
ISBN: 978-1-9822-5015-7 (hc)
ISBN: 978-1-9822-5016-4 (e)

Library of Congress Control Number: 2020911265

Balboa Press rev. date: 08/28/2020

To my parents, I owe you my amazing life
To my siblings, my forever rocks
To my beloved, you bless my life every day

*"I wish I can show you,
when you are lonely or in darkness,
the astonishing light of your own being."*

Hafiz

CONTENTS

FOREWORD

I met Rouba in May 2018 when she came to Florida to attend the Food Addiction Institute / ACORN Food Addiction Professional Training that I was leading. As a recovering food addict, Rouba was terrified of gaining back the weight she had lost. She came to the US all the way from the Middle East to gain a more solid understanding about food addiction recovery. I am delighted to witness the birth of this book. As millions of people grapple with obesity around the world, it is a personal testimony to the reality of overeating and the possibility of a sustainable recovery.

While many believe that eating less and exercising more is the solution to overeating, there is an increased body of evidence showing that a broader approach is needed. Food addiction is just like drug and alcohol addiction. Food addicts develop a chemical dependency in their brain to food, mainly sugar and flour, which impedes their ability to control their food intake. For about the 50% of obese people and 25% of overweight people that are food addicts, it does take much more than a diet and therapy to address their longstanding dependency on food.

Having worked with more than 4,000 middle and late stage food addicts for over twenty-five years, I can more than ascertain that diets alone don't work. Simple therapy alone does not work. What works for food addicts is surrender. Surrendering, through physical abstinence, the binge foods and abusive eating behaviors. Surrendering to rigorous honesty with all thoughts and feelings about food and developing the skills to cope with any feeling. Surrendering to whatever structure and support is needed. Ultimately, surrendering to the process of a spiritual experience. There is an endless number of spiritual paths that will work and I am happy that Rouba is sharing hers.

Through this book, Rouba illustrates her personal journey of overcoming overeating and how she has found a new balance in life. Readers will understand how to achieve a physical, emotional and spiritual balance in support of sustainable weight loss. I recommend this book to anyone struggling with a lifetime of overeating and eager to become healthy on a body, mind and spirit level.

Phil Werdell
Founder of the Food Addiction Institute

PREFACE

I have written this book to share a personal journey of recovery from food addiction. I struggled with weight all my life. I hid my shame, kept my head high and lived in my mind. All attempts to control my weight would fail. I had an old hunger inside: a deep hole that no amount of food could permanently fill. I compensated by being an accomplished girl.

Through this book, I explain that overeating is not the source of the problem but rather the consequence of a feeling of unease. I never chose to be fat. As a child, I would hide and rail against God for giving me a big appetite and an ugly body. I hated my body and just did not know what to do with it. Food comforted my constant restlessness. By acting as my magical tranquilizer, food helped me maintain the appearance of a seemingly composed, accomplished and well-behaved woman.

Then one day, while cycling through the Sri Lankan countryside, I fell and did not fully recover after the accident. At thirty-nine, I looked in the mirror and saw a fat, lonely and unhappy workaholic. My life looked great on paper, yet I was miserable. My body's rebellion triggered a mid-life crisis. So began my search for fullness outside of food.

By sharing my story, I am hoping to reach out to a wider audience of overeaters to help them understand the complexity of overeating and how recovery from food addiction involves a physical, emotional and spiritual transformation. As a healer and food addiction counselor, I illustrate a sustainable path to weight release built on addressing the unease within us.

This book is also addressed to overachieving women facing a mid-life crisis. By sharing my story of change and transformation, I hope to inspire readers that are struggling with direction. Change can look overwhelming given the uncertainties ahead, yet standing still is a license to being dead while alive. I share my journey of transition from an accomplished corporate leader to a novice healer.

ACKNOWLEDGEMENT

I offer my endless gratitude to Phil Werdell for being the first person to read my manuscript and give me constructive feedback. I had heard of Phil years before I met him, and I feel honored to have become a food addiction counselor under his guidance.

This book bears the touch of many beloved family members. Thank you Malak Kalmoni Chehab, my cousin, and Rania Odaymat, my one and only sister, for your editing contributions. I owe my brother Malek Chalabi the book cover design. Together with his wife Shirley Hendrickson, they helped me finalize the book title.

I would like to express my appreciation to all the change agents that participated in shaping my path from emptiness to fullness.

I was blessed to meet many catalysts in Dubai. Safa Zok, life coach and best friend, I can't thank you enough for making me believe in myself. I am indebted to Thetahealers Maya Badran and Tony Shoushani of Awakening the Masters, and to Elias Kanakri. I was able to shift perspectives thanks to the many courses I took with them. I am forever grateful to Dara El Ayed, from My Journey, my angel and guide in recovering from food addiction. Sometimes, the universe sends a pusher: Andrea Anstiss holds this honor, as she catalyzed my departure from an organized life and my adventure into the unknown, in addition to teaching me Reiki.

As I began my global pilgrimage, I encountered many wise teachers who supported me in my transition. Osho Afroz Meditation Center in Greece has a fond place in my heart. I was blessed to participate in a multitude of workshops provided by Satyarthi Peloquin and Sambhavo Lombardo of Path of Love, Svarup and Prematha of Primal Tantra, Kaifi of From Separation to Unity, and Nirupam Sufi Gyan. I owe my knowledge of body oriented healing modalities thanks to the Integral Body Institute in Poland. I did my Biodynamic Breathwork and Trauma Release training under the guidance of Giten Tonkov and Nisarga Dobosz. Thanks to Simon Calder, I learnt Qigong. I am forever grateful to Prema McKeever for her teachings on trauma. Finally, thanks to Gisele Seto and Rami AbouJawdeh, who thought me Thai Yoga Massage in Lebanon. I wouldn't be the healer I am today without all the wisdom and inspiration they passed on to me.

LETTER TO MY YOUNGER SELF

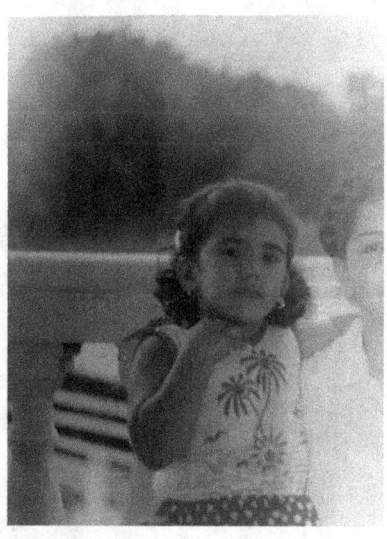

I write this letter to you as I turn forty-three today. I so wish I could hug you right now and make you feel the love this universe has for you. I wish I could make you see how beautiful you are in the eyes of the creator. You are going to become an amazing girly girl, unapologetically yourself, a free independent woman. You are going to live a life of exploration and adventure, a life of carefree timelessness, taking your time to enjoy every moment. Rest assured, you are deeply loved. Each cell of your body is overflowing with the love of your family, friends, and the many angels that keep coming your way. Your big heart will continue to shine spreading love everywhere. I can't get enough of looking into your beautiful eyes. You are going to fall in love with yourself and reach a state of peace, playfulness and joy. You are going to live again with your mommy and hug each other every day. And by the way, you will keep on drawing the coconut tree on your T-shirt. My sweet beloved, I want you to feel safe. Trust that life will bring what is in your highest and best interest. Don't allow others to make you feel small. Listen to your intuition. It's the voice of your truth. Relax my love. You are safe. Forever Yours!

Posted on Instagram on July 4, 2019

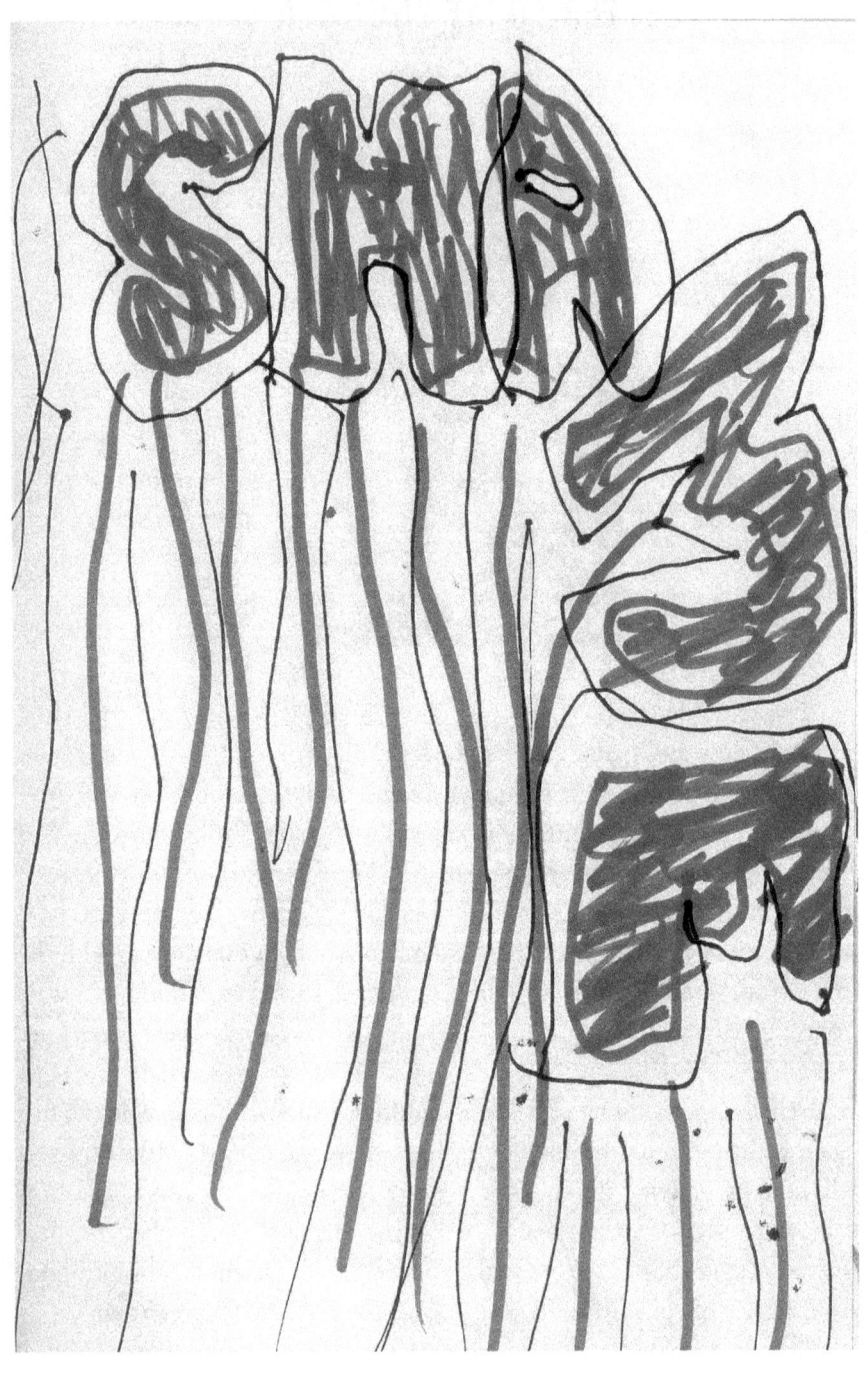

CHAPTER 1

GROWING UP WITH SHAME

■

Neurotic shame is at the root and fuel of all compulsive and addictive behavior... The drivenness in any addiction is about the ruptured self, the belief that one is flawed as a person.

- John Bradshaw

I came to life on Sunday July 4, 1976 at five o'clock in the morning at the beginning of Lebanon's civil war, in the Northern city of Tripoli. I was a second child to Mohamad and Faten, two years younger than my sister Rania. Mom was nineteen years old and dad thirty-seven, at the time. Water and electricity were permanently cut off the week I was born. Roads were closed and Israeli jets were hovering low. Together as a family, we escaped to Ghana, in West Africa, and joined the rest of my mom's family, who had been established there for three generations. I was one month old then, and throughout my life, I would feel fortunate to have grown up in a peaceful country surrounded by uncles, aunts and cousins.

My experience of my beginning is quite different from my mother's story of a low maintenance baby who was very easy to please. Unknowingly to all of us, the infant in me had sensed the war and interpreted the family's stressors as a rejection. I began my life feeling unwelcome. I would often get inundated by a sensation of poison spreading through my blood. My skin would itch and burn. I would feel the need to disappear. I calmed down through isolation, eating and sleep. I compensated by becoming a well-behaved girl who was accomplished at school. Peace came through living under the radar and attracting the least attention possible.

Mom was selfless, in the true Lebanese Mediterranean tradition. She had little life of her own, and totally devoted herself to our upbringing.

Because she left school at sixteen to get married, our education was her highest priority. She communicated her love through cooking and acts of service. Dad was not involved in the every day matters of our family. Mom was the one in charge. Emotional expression was absent. We never hugged nor kissed. Crying was not allowed. No matter what happened, I always felt it was my fault. I swallowed all my discomforts and never sought help. I did not want to be a burden to my parents who were usually sad and overwhelmed. After all, a good girl is strong.

School was my refuge. To date, my heart is filled with the loving presence of all the teachers and administrators of the Ecole Francaise d'Accra, a small French school of about 250 students in the Roman Ridge neighborhood of Accra in Ghana. The French principal Mr. Ducamp knew all of the students by name. I felt seen, loved and appreciated for my individuality. To me, school felt like a true home. I thrived. I was armed with a curious mind, and my pursuit of knowledge and learning was endless. My mind felt infinite in contrast with the awkwardness of my body. Excelling at school came with ease. I enjoyed the status of the accomplished, which made both of my parents proud.

I was a sad girl. I remember teachers telling mom: "She's the ideal student. If only she would smile." I still hear echoes of mom's nagging voice: "Smile... Stop frowning... Straighten your back..." Those expectations took so much effort. Over time, I learned to wear a mask and mastered the art of the fake smile. Deep inside, I did not know how to be happy. Life felt heavy. Giggly people irritated me. Whenever I tried to play and let go, an inner voice would warn me: *Don't get distracted. Stay alert, something bad is about to happen.* I simply did not know how to have fun.

Food was my friend. I had a love affair with sweets. Mom was always baking something for someone. I would salivate at the smell. When I started eating her cakes and cookies, I had to finish them all. While I consciously knew I should not eat so much, I just could not stop. Mom was constantly troubled by my overeating and began hiding sweets. That made me feel rejected. Why did she hate me? I would go on treasure hunts while she was asleep and secretly eat everything. I enjoyed witnessing her embarrassment when she would have guests and realize there was nothing left to serve them. I felt victorious. I longed for her love. Food was her expression. Yet, she refused to feed me. She loved her guests and the rest of the family but did not love me. Eating was my silent revenge: *Those cookies are mine!*

My body was my enemy. I remember hiding and railing against God for giving me a big appetite and an ugly body. Mom would point out how beautiful other girls were and comment: "It's a pity; you're so smart." I did not fit her vision of what a daughter's physique should look like. I hated my body. If only I could disappear. I aggressed it through eating. I survived by escaping to my mind. By dissociating from my body, I could live in partial denial of my pain. I became my mind.

I dreamt of being an independent and successful superwoman, free from the limitations of a husband and children. I did not want to be a boring and naive married woman. My mom, aunts and their friends had mostly married precociously and were totally dependent on their husbands, brothers, fathers and children. I dreamt of living life on my own terms. This hope for a better future gave me the energy to keep going. For now, I was stuck. Through sleep, I escaped the prison every day. When it was too much, I would go to bed early and exit this world. I felt free. Sleep gave me a break and the energy to return to life and face a new day.

I began dieting at thirteen in the hope of fitting society's expectation of what a girl's body should look like. After all, "a woman's worth is in her looks". I limited my food intake for some time, yet I could not sustain the torture. I was constantly hungry. Eating was my favorite activity. Food calmed my nerves, gave me pleasure and made the actual moment livable. While I consciously knew I should not eat so much, I just could not stop. Food was my fuel, my energizer, my tranquilizer, and my abusive lover. We had a love-hate relationship. I just could not live without eating as I wished. Food thoughts dominated my mind with ongoing inner fights about whether to eat or not to eat. I would succeed in silencing this voice and taming this hunger for a few months and then one day, it would just explode out of me at a higher intensity. My weight was like a yo-yo, with the ups consistently higher than the downs. I felt imprisoned in my body, trapped in the family, and stuck in my life. That caused me to eat even more and gain further weight.

Studying remained my focus after returning to Lebanon at the age of fifteen. It was 1991 and the civil war in Lebanon had just ended. We moved back to Tripoli, my parents' hometown. I struggled to find my place at the Lycee Franco-Libanais. Most of my classmates had been together at school since kindergarten. The war had bonded them. I suffocated in the sameness of an isolated society that had just begun to open up. I felt out of place. At home, we all struggled to adapt to a new life in Lebanon. Money was tight. I buried myself at home studying, in the hope of receiving a university scholarship. I did not participate in any after-school activities. Eating seemed to be my only hobby. On the day of my high school mandatory sports exam, I promised myself to never exercise again. I was done with sports.

While I had witnessed the immense sacrifices of my parents and extended family in setting me up for success, I was so relieved to leave the house and move to another city to study at the American University of Beirut (AUB). I was blessed by a scholarship from the Hariri Foundation. AUB's beautiful campus became my home. I was now free! Thankfully, my parents gave me space to experience life. I majored in economics while taking all my elective courses in political science. I had a passion for both and was fascinated by the rise and fall of nations. I lived on campus at the Murex women's dormitories and spent my free time there supported by a group of fellow women. I wish the walls could speak and replay all those beautiful memories of us crammed in my friend Hala's room, chit chatting about life.

During my time at AUB, Lebanon was beginning to reconstruct after fifteen years of civil war. It was the mid-nineties. There was a feeling of hope about a better future. AUB was a melting pot with students from all regions and backgrounds. I thrived in this micro-cosmos of Lebanese society in all its sectarian, regional and economic diversity. I did not have to fit in. I could just be myself. I felt free in this openness.

Run Run

Faster

Faster

Faster

Run Run

Faster

Faster

Run Run

CHAPTER 2

BECOMING A FAT WORKAHOLIC

■

Don't seek happiness. If you seek it, you won't find it, because seeking is the antithesis of happiness.

- Eckhart Tolle

I began working full time at the age of twenty-one while most of my friends pursued higher degrees. My family needed financial support. I did not have time to waste. While my parents did not have the connections needed to land me a job, I benefited from an unfortunate situation at the Ministry of Economy and Trade. The project manager and a few of her staff had suddenly resigned, and the minister's team was keen on immediately filling in three positions. I got the job without knowing anyone there, and was now in a position to earn an income to support my family.

Being overweight, I was self-conscious about my physical appearance. I felt I did not look good enough. I compensated through extreme hard work. My first two years of career were a learning curve about the dysfunctional Lebanese state. I worked in a United Nations funded project that attracted talent into a parallel government administration to fill the gap wherever the civil service was failing. My job was to provide trade information to foreign organizations eager to do business with Lebanon. I would also support the Minister's office with miscellaneous research requests. I loved absorbing a wealth of complex information, analyzing it and then presenting it in simplified ways. Those were the early days of e-mail. There was no internet and no Google. Getting information involved talking to people and reviewing laws and regulations. I enjoyed being the nice accomplished girl, and embraced any additional task with open arms.

Now that I was earning my own money, I began going out more often and discovered Beirut beyond the walls of the university. Together with my high school friend Sana, I joined the Rotaract Club of Beirut. As Ghandi would say: *"The best way to find yourself is to loose yourself in the service of others."* I felt needed and took positions of responsibility in Rotaract and later Rotary. I enjoyed managing all aspects of the club, especially the educational and community projects. I felt inspired by many role models, and became more outgoing.

After the Ministry, I spent seven years at the American Embassy, influencing economic and business policies in Lebanon. I loved the world of diplomacy, and enjoyed being in the corridors of power, making and shaping policies with all of the paradoxes that entail. The American work environment emboldened the woman in me. As a Lebanese woman, I was raised to shrink myself and play small. At the Embassy, I learnt to shine.

I began to experience deep emptiness in my mid-twenties despite all my professional success. My friends and flat mates were getting married and building families while I was still single. I was fat and ugly and struggled to compete with other women. I felt unattractive to men. Shopping for clothes was a painful reminder of my heavy body, and of the impossibility of finding something that would be both comfortable and flattering. I would buy expensive clothes and accessories in the hope of looking good, and to compensate for my lack of looks. I felt empty. The hole inside me kept growing and no food, accomplishment or acquisition could fill it. I discovered yoga and began exercising, after being physically inactive for six years. Yoga was soft and allowed me to reconnect with my body. I especially enjoyed the candle meditation at the end of the class. It calmed me down.

Food was my escape. I loved gourmet food and was always on the lookout for the best culinary experience. I would always favor family sharing style to distract others from the large quantities I ate. I hated vegetables and gravitated towards lots of desserts. I would often eat in hiding or in the car as I could not wait to get home. Thanks to supportive and loving colleagues and family, I embarked on a high carbs low fat diet together with my high school friend Fida. We both lost around fifteen kilograms (around thirty-three pounds). We felt great. I began exercising more and swam multiple times a week for a whole year. My body looked good for a short while. Little by little, however, I regained the lost weight.

Being thin did not address my deep need to feel seen and loved, nor my feeling of emptiness.

I felt a longing to do more with my life. I was bored at work and could not imagine myself working at the Embassy until retirement like everyone else. I was constantly restless. Being a public face came at a personal price. People in society were either overly friendly in anticipation of a service I could offer them, or aggressive as a reaction to US policy in Israel and Iraq at that time. The July Israeli war in 2006 shook me to my core. Lebanon's trajectory had been going downhill since 2004 in the run up to Prime Minister Hariri's assassination. Making a difference for my country became difficult. The sheer extent of the destruction made me feel powerless, humiliated and inferior. I was done with public work but had no clue what to do next.

Two career transition books *Through the Brick Wall* and *What Color Is Your Parachute* came to my rescue. They had been in my bookshelf since a trip to New York City five years earlier. I began reading to get distracted from the unrest. I enjoyed occupying my mind, and felt productive amidst all the destruction and misery. By the end of the stalemate, I had developed a roadmap for my career transition. My friend from university Sarah and an ex-colleague Guy helped me revamp my resume.

Rather than asking people for a job, I intended to individually sit with a handful of successful people and brainstorm together about potential career opportunities. I reached out to Walid, a prominent lawyer who had worked across continents. We had developed a special work relationship over the years. I valued his wisdom. As we discussed what I could possibly do, he matched my skills with a public affairs position that had been hard to fill by a mutual contact, Fady. I had never planned to hold a career in public affairs and did not know such a profession existed until Walid saw my potential. Thankfully, Fady was quick to hire me after the July war had ended. After nine years of government work, I moved to the private sector to work for a multinational pharmaceutical company. At times I wondered: *What am I doing among pharmacists and doctors?* While my medical knowledge was limited to the biology classes I took in high school, my knowhow of how governments operated was a much-needed skill.

My attempts to loose weight continued. I had diet meals delivered to my doorstep for two years. I had liposuction. I also tried paleo. I would loose a good amount of weight only to regain it when my stress levels peaked. Then a few years later, I would somehow motivate myself to go on a new diet, only to regain the lost weight a few months down the line and add on even more kilos/pounds. I was perplexed by how others managed to stay thin and not me. There was so much hunger in me: a sense of emptiness that kept eating away at my insides. I began exercising more. I hired personal trainers who put me on a stringent exercise regimen. While I experienced improvements in my fitness level, I just could not sustain it beyond a year. Movement took so much effort. It felt like I was moving mountains. I wanted to be still, and in thinking mode.

An MBA mid-career gave me the confidence to become more daring. By then, I held a regional role that involved frequent travel. I would often travel to countries within Europe and the Middle East, and became exposed to the bigger business world. The security situation in Lebanon was deteriorating due to random assassinations and bombings that would happen every few weeks. Dubai seemed like an interesting work location, yet I had no clue how to get a job there. The opportunity came thanks to a peer from another company. We were both speakers at a government conference in Jordan. One day, he called me sharing two vacancies in Dubai, although I had not yet verbalized to anyone my interest in leaving Lebanon. He was God sent, since I was eager for a change.

I relocated to Dubai in 2010. That was the beginning of a major shift. Dubai is a land of opportunities of the modern world. Unlike Lebanon's self-destructive energy, Dubai has an expansive momentum where dreams become a reality. There were no limits to what was possible. Life was smooth with no distractions other than working non-stop and frequent business travel. The work environment was quite intense. Competition was cutthroat. As a regional hub for Africa and the Middle East, work possibilities were endless. There was no ceiling to what could be achieved. I covered regions as wide as Africa, the Middle East and Asia all the way to Australia. Business travel provided me with a wide exposure to the world. I loved this enrichment and empowerment of my abilities. I missed family and friends, yet was relieved from the social pressure that my Lebanese culture imposed on me.

I strongly identified with my work identity. It gave me a great sense of worthiness. I felt needed. I took duties seriously and over-delivered by overextending myself. Work came first, above my personal life. I was self-driven and did not need motivation. Everything was under control. I was always one step ahead, prepared with a backup plan B and C just in case. I hated compliments and would try to change the topic of the conversation, as it made me feel like a fraud. As I evolved in my career, promotions, awards, salary raises, new jobs gave me a sense of fulfillment. Yet, I still felt that something was lacking, and that I needed to work harder. Somehow, my list of accomplishments would go back to zero at midnight, and I needed to prove myself all over again the next day.

My career trajectory was unplanned. While other friends evolved within the same organization, I moved from the government sector to an Embassy, then shifted to the private sector, worked in the pharmaceutical and food industries, creating strategies of engagement with government and civil society. My work scope expanded over time into communication and crisis management. Each time my learning curve flattened, I would spiral into an existential crisis that would push me into making a new leap. For my inner conqueror, moving on was a matter of survival. Once I had set my intention on 'what's next', opportunities would present themselves to me seemingly by coincidence, thanks to people I had met along the way and their belief in my potential.

But no matter what I did, I just could not be happy. I thought when my life became more organized, I would become happy, or happier at the very least. Somehow, there was always something more that I needed to do to reach that happiness goal : that extra accomplishment at work, a more senior role, a higher salary, or making my parents happy. I became a Vice President of Corporate Affairs at the age of thirty-eight. I was over the moon. I had made it, or so I thought.

The peak is a lonely place. I covered multiple markets on different time zones and workweeks. Travel was frequent. Work was non-stop, day, night, weekends and holidays. I became isolated from friends and family. I felt very much like a wind-up doll with a dysfunctional turnkey. On paper, my life looked great; people believed I had it all. In reality, I was miserable. I was drowning at work, yet few in my personal life could understand what was happening.

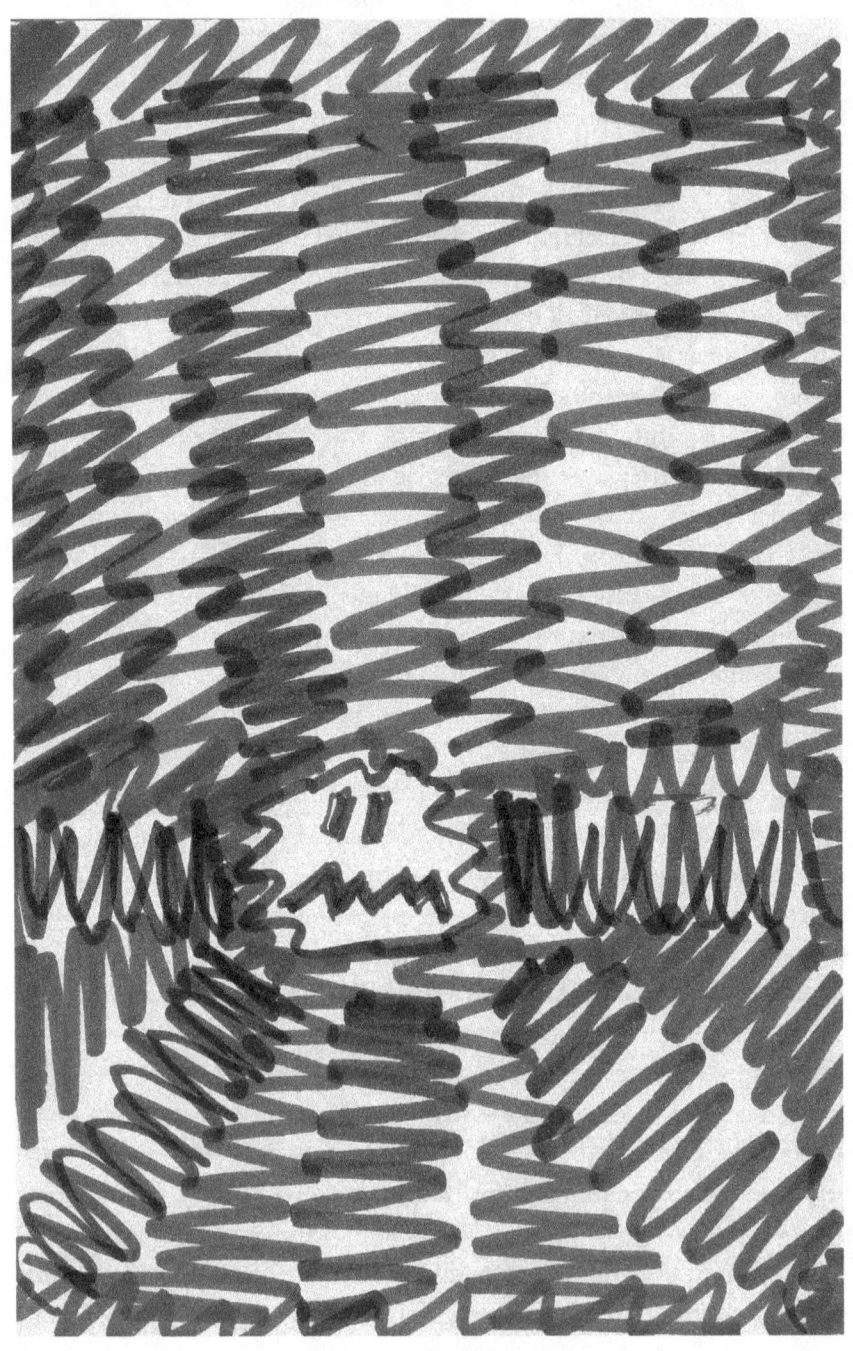

My big hidden hole

CHAPTER 3

WHEN MY BODY SAID NO

■

Incredible change happens in your life when you decide to take control of what you have power over instead of craving control over what you don't.

- Steve Maraboli

As part of a company restructuring, I was pressured to take on a smaller role. *How could this be possible after such hard work? I had given my all to my career.* I was fluctuating between denial and anger. At the age of forty, I came to a painful realization: *I was a fat unmarried workaholic who was a cash machine. Work and family were taking advantage of me.*

I escaped to Sri Lanka in the midst of all this confusion for an express forty-eight hour trip to cycle through the countryside. That meant travelling overnight on Thursday, cycling on Friday and Saturday, then flying back overnight on Saturday so I could work on Sunday. That was my pace then: travelling at night to win time, and then putting up with long days. Slowing down was not an option.

I crashed after a long day of cycling. The bicycle bumped into a hole and flipped upside down, smashing my face to the ground and causing a wound above my left eyebrow. To make things worse, my maternal grandmother died that day. I could barely lift my head up, and had to stay in bed for the next few days. My body was forced to shut down. Everything changed afterwards. I felt like a leaking tank with many holes. Less work and more family time did not help. Whatever I did, I would regain my energy shortly, only to loose it the minute I stepped back into the office. Work seemed to be sapping all of my positive energy.

A colleague sensed my suffering and suggested that I try Thetahealing, a healing technique that identifies the beliefs that bind your growth, and that empowers you to live life with positive thoughts. I could not really understand what it involved, but I was nevertheless eager to experiment, as I felt out of options. Two days later, I had my first one-on-one session with Thetahealer Maya Badran and experienced calming vibrations through each cell of my body. My mind, body and spirit felt like they were getting closer. Over the long and hot Dubai summer, my attention began to shift inwards. I was spending more time at home and began to befriend myself. A new romance was born between my outer and inner self, bringing with it a sense of magical intimacy. I could not wait to be back home each night to cook and have a long bath; to just be there with myself. I was calmer.

After the summer, I wanted more of this healing feeling and began attending Thetahealing courses on weekends together with my friend Amelle. Surrounded by a community of people with no masks, I realized I was not alone in my suffering. Many were similarly passing through a crisis of some sort. We were all there in our naked truth, exploring a new approach to becoming centered through meditation and prayer.

My vision of reality began to shift. My mind was slowly loosing its grip on me, as my consciousness kept expanding. I would close my eyes and pay attention to my inner silence. The shy voice of my intuition awoke, sending me funny messages that were not necessarily aligned with the logic and precision of my mind. As I developed trust in my intuition, I was able to lower the volume and intensity of my mind. I became less controlling of outcomes, and more open to life and possibilities.

I made my peace with God. We could finally communicate directly in free form, anywhere, anytime without a religious intermediary or a prayer format. I loved this direct link. My faith in life increased. I felt supported, and no longer needed to carry all the heavy burdens on my own. I felt connected to the rest of the universe. I was an integral part of this universe, and all of our energies were interconnected.

Happiness came to me in small things. Author Elizabeth Gilbert inspired me to create a gratitude jar, where I would often write myself little notes. Life became playful. I would wake up in the morning and decide to live today as the first day of my life, approaching every small thing with the curiosity and excitement of a beginner. Other days, I would live today as the last day, celebrating every bit of urgency. I started doing random acts of kindness such as allowing a car to pass while driving, or looking into the eyes of a sad looking stranger and smiling. Their reactions filled my heart with so much joy. On dull days, I would challenge myself to do something new. Creativity comes to the clueless, bringing a fresh perspective to doing the same old thing. On bad days, I would say "Cheers!" and set my intention on it being the best day of my life. The universe never disappointed, as I felt that the greater my optimism, the better the outcome of my day. There was always something unexpected that made it special all on its own.

Through Thetahealing, I began a process of forgiveness. Rather than wait for others to forgive me, I took my power back and embarked on forgiving them instead. Nelson Mandela says: *"Resentment is like drinking poison and then hoping it will kill your enemies."* Forty years of poison were eating me up, creating tensions in my relationships and dis-ease in my body. So, I began to forgive others with my own process and without their participation, with no expectation that there would be any apologies. I would write a letter and then imagine the person facing me, while I addressed him or her. Thankfully, a fellow Thetahealer would hold my hand and support me through the difficult undertaking.

Forgiveness is not a straightforward journey. Sometimes, it was instantaneous, while other times, I had to work on it multiple times to achieve success. Occasionally, I thought I had forgiven, only to realize months later that it was not the case. More forgiveness was needed. Once I was able to identify the positive things that came about despite the hurt, I was able to move forward and shift from a perspective of pain to a perspective of blessing. Perceiving the gift behind the trauma was not obvious, as murky emotions kept interfering with my vision. It took time for my healing process to evolve.

After about six months of forgiveness work, I began experiencing a shift in my relationship with my mother. It became lighter and more playful. While she was not directly involved in my process, her approach towards me changed when I changed. It did not happen in one go. I came to discover months later that she had been feeling increasingly guilty of all the pain she had indirectly caused me, but she would still try to brush it off rather than discuss it, or resolve it. I knew none of the pain she had inflicted was intentional. After all, she had done her best, and yet I still struggled with her denial. Then one day, many months after I had forgiven her, we had an argument and she acknowledged my pain. All I needed from her by that point was her acknowledgement, which in itself was a breakthrough. The rest of the people I have forgiven have not apologized, but I did not expect them to. By forgiving them, I freed myself from their poison.

I still needed to forgive myself though. Over the years, I had become the queen of endurance, mastering the art of accommodation and adaptation to all kinds of situations no matter how challenging they were. I took pride in being the hard working, drama free woman. This came with a heavy price tag and a lot of extra weight. I started connecting with anger. I was angry for having put all my hopes and wishes in the work basket. I was angry for having neglected myself. I was angry for enduring abuse and not expressing my rage about it. I was livid at myself for placing others' wellbeing above my own. I was no longer willing to compromise on this front and was, now, ready to put myself first.

I began to cry during healing sessions. I did not know how to cry, given that crying was forbidden in my upbringing. At first, crying felt like the violent explosion of a volcano, leaving me with a headache that would persist for days. It got smoother with time. I became lighter and was able to switch back to my normal self faster after an outburst.

I came to understand what led me to this place of crisis. The workaholic facade was a cover for my shame. Deep inside, I felt unworthy, so I earned society's respect by becoming an accomplished executive. I no longer had any stamina for pushing and forcing life into a specific definition of success. Through the accident, my body told me: *Enough!* I finally listened and began taking care of myself through focusing on areas that I had direct control over: my health and wellbeing.

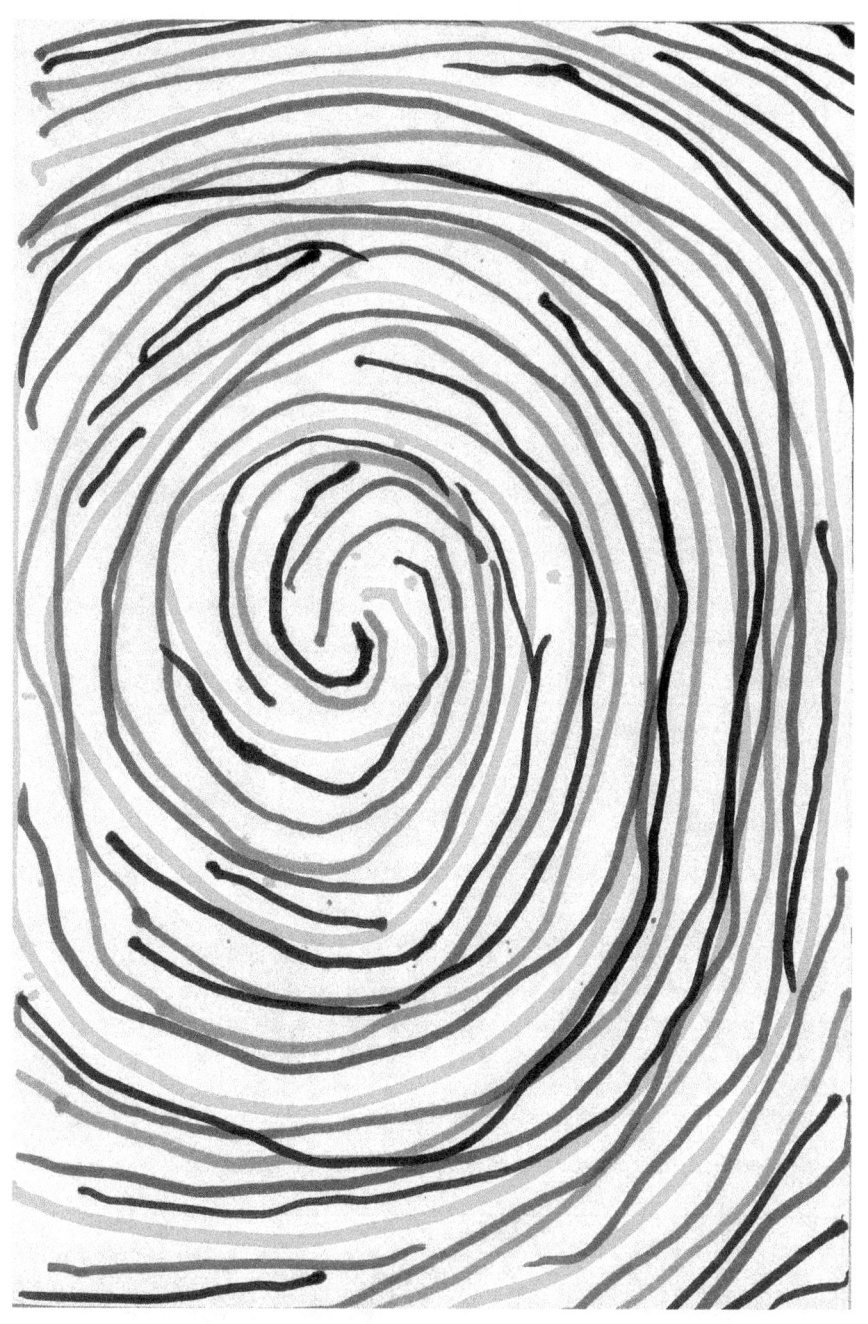

When life begins to expand

CHAPTER 4

LOVING THE ENEMY

■

And God said, love your enemy, and I obeyed him and
loved myself.

- Gibran Khalil Gibran

I had been eating three chocolate bars a day for months. I worked
at a chocolate factory, and there was chocolate at every meeting, lounge,
and desk. After six months of Thetahealing, I began to question my
relationship with food. God sensed my readiness and made me bump into
Nadia. Her weight-loss transformation gave me the push to stop body
aggression and begin applying kindness.

The food addiction recovery program was my new-year's gift. Nadia
had explained that it was a special program with a two-day kick off
workshop, weekly meetings, and a WhatsApp group. It sounded like the
kind of support I needed. The facilitator for the program, Dara El Ayed,
was not a dietician. She was a recovering food addict. I was attracted by
this concept of being guided through a process by someone who had
experienced it. That was quite a contrast from dieticians who were never
fat, too perfect, and seemed to be condescending in their treatment of any
transgression.

During the kickoff weekend, I started to understand the nature of
my food addiction. Unlike emotional eaters, my brain had a chemical
dependency on food, particularly sugar and flour. I was now getting to
understand that I had an irritated nervous system that demanded instant
comfort. When parents are not emotionally available to support children
in learning how to calm down, children begin to search for substitutes to
regulate their nervous system. A neglected child shuts down her pain by
stopping to feel. In this state of emotional starvation, the child seeks relief

elsewhere. In my case, I chose food. I had a mental obsession with food and an incessant urge to eat. My brain triggered a feeling of false hunger. Food would come to its rescue providing the immediate high it needed. I was addicted to food the same way an alcoholic is addicted to booze. For all those years, I thought I lacked a strong will. I now realized I was like a car with dysfunctional breaks: when I started eating, I just could not stop.

The food addiction recovery model gave me hope as it addressed my physical, emotional and spiritual needs, while mending the disconnectedness I had experienced between my mind, body and soul. Traditional diets focusing on eating discipline and routine had failed me. I was now eager to approach my relationship with food differently, by working through this program. A fellow recovering food addict, Aya, inspired me to put myself first. Indeed, I had been fueling myself with food in order to take care of everyone. I had to now place myself first, because in all honesty that was the only thing within my span of control.

As per the twelve steps of Alcoholics Anonymous, any successful recovery from addiction is anchored in surrender. I first perceived this surrender as a failure, very much like becoming a defeated soldier. And yet, there was so much freedom in resigning from my self-acclaimed position of CEO of the universe. I was dissatisfied with where I was in life. I came to an epiphany: *How about I relax and allow life to surprise me?* I willfully stopped pushing and forcing life in a certain direction, and allowed God to take charge. Since I was no longer running the show, I could use this spare energy to take care of myself.

Anchored in self-love, I was now going to remove sugar and flour from my life, not forever though, just one day at a time. Each meal, I will choose not to eat them. I started having four portion-controlled meals a day. I would eat home-prepared unprocessed foods, and fast in-between meals. Unknowingly, I was embarking on a radical lifestyle change, where food would no longer be my go-to tranquilizer.

I started eating more vegetables. I struggled at first and soon got bored of eating tomatoes, eggplants and zucchinis. That's when I began experimenting with new vegetables. My rule was I would make a judgment after three consecutive trials. Ninety percent of vegetables passed that test. My taste buds changed as I stopped eating refined and processed foods. I could now taste the individual flavor of each vegetable, and began to love their rawness. I fell in love with bell peppers, cabbage, cauliflower, and all types of greens.

As my body cleared of sugar and flour, I began to have less food thoughts. My mind was no longer consumed with the constant inner fight: *I want to eat!, No, Yes, I am going to eat now! No!* I loved this peace of mind. My body became more communicative. I could feel the impact of the food I was consuming. Raw food energized me. Cooked food made my body warmer on cold days. I struggled to digest some beans, so I cut them out of my diet. I loved this direct feedback and it helped me adjust my food choices; even my skin color changed. Obviously, my body was now composed of fruits and vegetables rather than refined sugar and flour.

I became the queen of planning and organization. Every day, I spent an hour and a half in the kitchen preparing my meals and packing them in ready-to-go containers. My friend, Ghada, would joke about my moving fridge; however, I did not have to worry about what to eat when I was out. I always had my food with me. While I ate my meals at work, I was thankful for this special person taking care of me. I was blessed by the love of my inner cook. I would freeze many meals for those days when I would come back from business trips. I even found an online delivery service for fruits and vegetables. I would order while travelling and then find the box by my doorstep as I arrived from the airport.

This food program was much more than a diet. I was relearning how to understand my body. Whenever I was hungry, I began exploring the emotions behind my false hunger: *Am I tired? Have I been resting enough? How was my sleep the night before? Am I spending too much time outside of the house?* I would check my answers, and identify the reason behind my hunger. *Had anyone upset me? Had anything happened over the past days that I had ignored?* Many times, within forty-eight hours, I would remember an incident that had annoyed me in the past day or so. These are typically events that I tended to unconsciously sweep underneath the rug and erase from my awareness. Fear is another important emotion that I would scan for. I felt like the mother of a newborn baby learning to understand the needs of her infant and exploring what brings her child to a happily contented rhythm.

Thanks to Lana, I discovered a book by Louise Hay, *You Can Heal Your Life,* which has an index of psycho-somatic factors underlying any disease. If you pay close attention to the word it's: dis-ease, a lack of ease. I would look up what was physically bothering me and reflect about the insights the book was offering. We are made of energy, and it's crazy how negative beliefs activate pain in our body.

I became an expert in non-food activities. Friends would joke that going out with me kept them thin. Rather than eating out, I would meet a friend for a walking conversation. I would go out to cultural activities. I took voice coaching classes with lovely ex-opera singer, Renata, two evenings a week. I loved singing. It made me feel lighter, and relieved my stress after a long day of work. I discovered sound meditations. I would lie down and relax while a facilitator played various instruments, whose vibrations were interpreted by my body as love.

I was blessed by a community of warrior angels. Under Dara's leadership, we would meet on a weekly basis, share our struggles, and support each other on this new path of food freedom. This journey is in no way a clear-cut process. There were ups and downs, impasses, valleys and volcanoes. My only constant was my commitment to taking life one moment at a time, and doing what was necessary to care for myself in my moments of need.

I lost thirty kilograms (sixty-three pounds) within eighteen months. My body just kept shrinking. Any time I happened to look at it, I would do a double take: it did not feel like it was mine. Occasionally, I would be terrified. My mind would play games: *What if I were sick and dying?* However, I was mostly ecstatic. Here I was, at the age of fort-one, thinner than in my teenage years. I felt good, being in this new body. I enjoyed not having to squeeze myself into socially acceptable clothes that locked me up. I could now take as much breath and space as I wanted. That's quite a relief. Forty years of constant squeezing had made me feel restless, depressed, and imprisoned in this human body. I now felt as light as a bird. I hired a stylist and started dressing differently. I went back to horseback riding and cycling.

Growing up overweight, I had imagined that my life would be beautiful once I became slim. After a short period of euphoria, I came to realize that it was not that simple. Overeating is not the source of the problem but rather the consequence of a deep unease with life. My unease was still alive and kicking, even after I had stopped using food as a tranquilizer.

While I had achieved my dream of being slim, I was still far from the finish line. As a matter of fact, I was just embarking on a life long journey of inner connection and alignment with my body and soul's rhythm. This is where I had failed in the past: taking my excess weight at face value, and consequently seeing discipline as the answer to a diet. Unfortunately, this is also where many dieticians fail today. A big number of overeaters resort to surgery in the hope of rationing their food intake, only to slowly gain back the weight over a period of about five years. My journey had to take me on a path to genuine self-love: *my body is no longer my enemy, it is what I truly treasure the most.* My actions became grounded in this love connection. Overeaters are obsessed with food and confuse it with love. They are terrified of loosing their abusive lover.

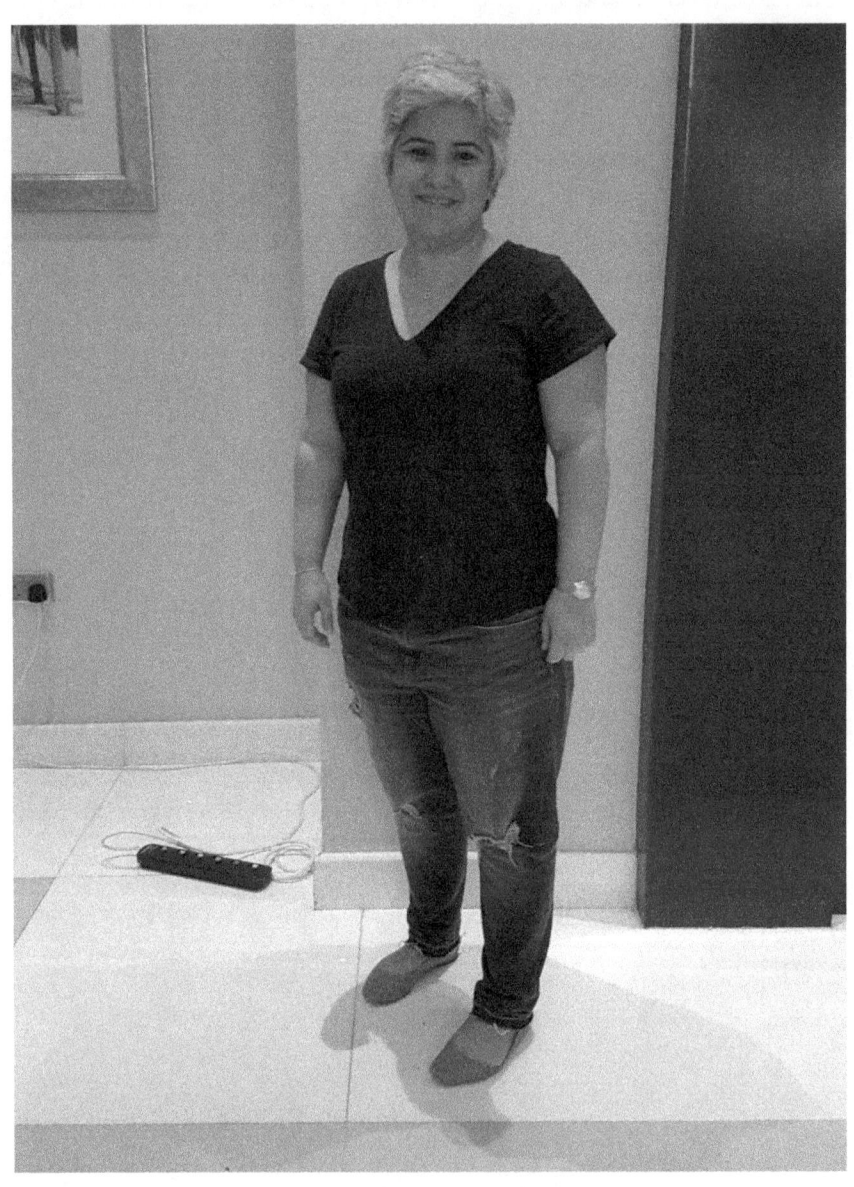

On my first day of food addiction recovery

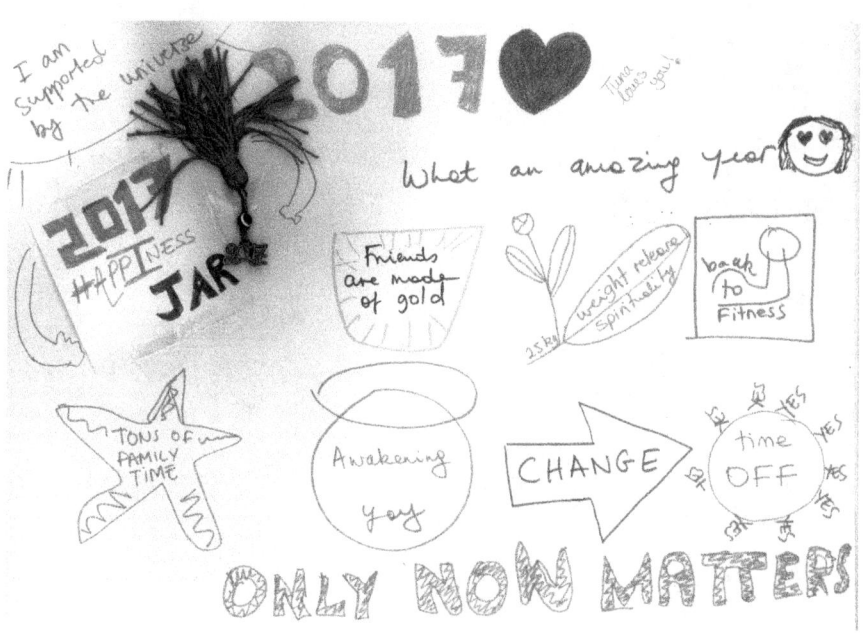

A summary of my 2017 happiness jar

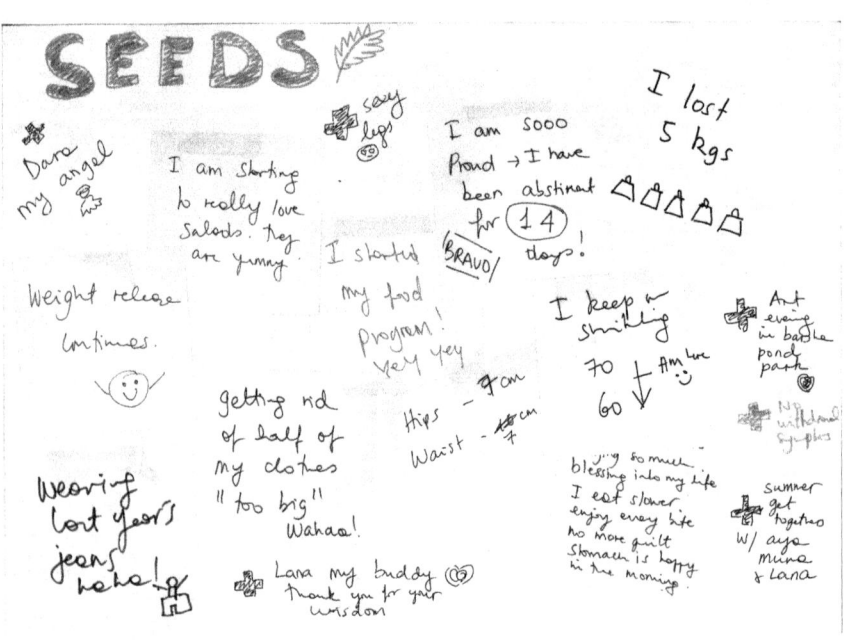

Happiness jar notes on Seeds, my food addiction recovery support group

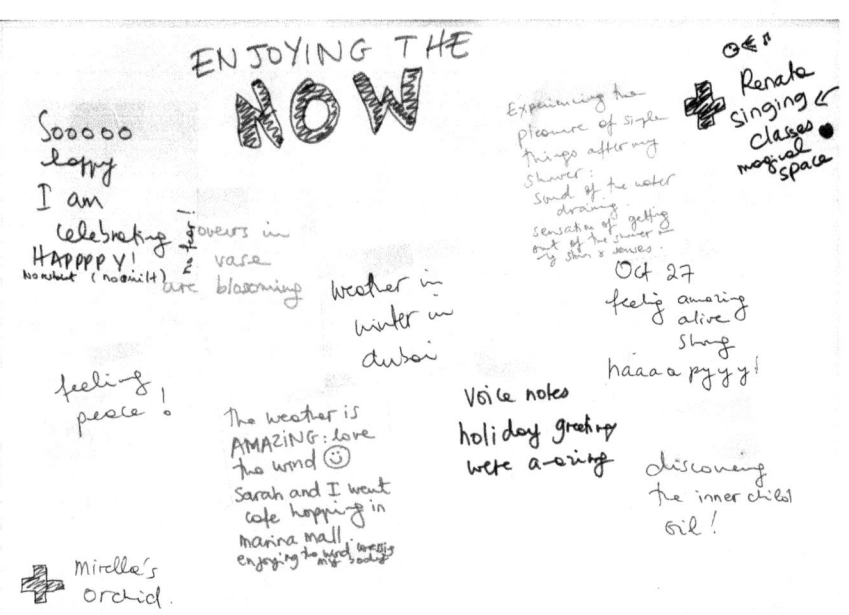

Notes from my happiness jar

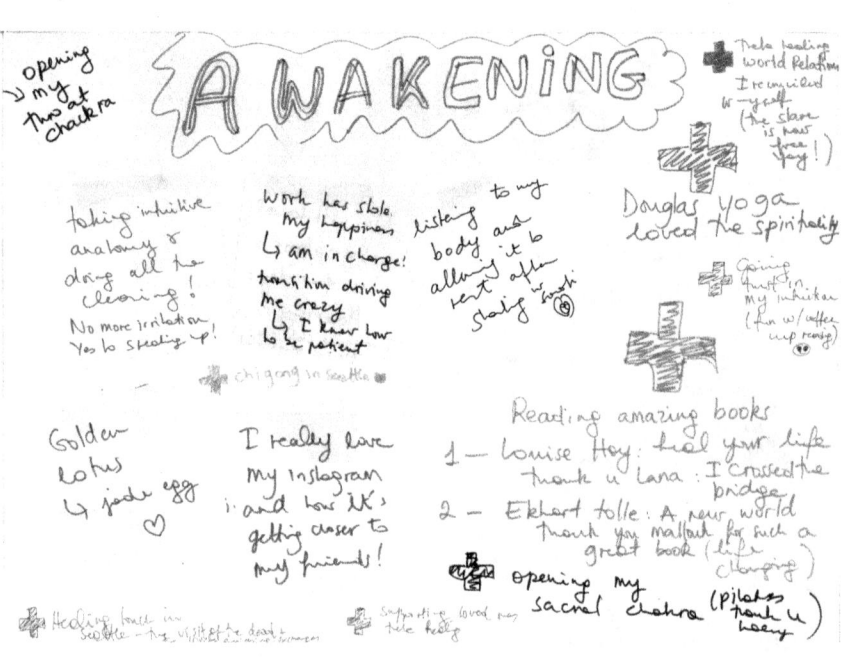

Notes from my happiness jar

■

THE UNKNOWN

Shake, shake, stability
Hello possibility!
Hello Mystery!
I welcome your discovery.
Thank you surprise,
For every moment you arise!
Let's dance Mr. Unknown,
Where the beauty of life is sown.
Together we flow,
Towards a horizon that makes me grow.

■

CHAPTER 5

JUMPING INTO THE UNKNOWN

■

And the day came when the risk to remain tight in a bud
was more painful than the risk it took to blossom.

- Anais Nin

Work felt like living on an island that is constantly on fire. We were
facing a variety of company restructurings that would lead to possible
layoffs. I had been moved into a new role that I was not enjoying. Over
the past year, I kept running away from the fire engulfing the workplace
only to find myself facing a cliff. I was afraid to jump. I would turn around
and walk back, convincing myself that the fire was not that bad. And there
I went, back and forth. I felt imprisoned on an island, too afraid to leave,
and yet too scared to embrace the necessary change.

My good friend and personal life coach, Safa, had suggested a year
earlier that I quit my job as it was only going to further impede my positive
progress. I resigned, but was persuaded by the company to stay on because
I was essential. That was exactly what I needed then: reassurance as to my
importance. A year later, I had a greater degree of awareness of the big price
that my health had paid in order to survive this fire. Something had to
give, but I was still terrified. At times, my fear was paralyzing. I remember
Tony Shoushani's voice, my first Thetahealing instructor repeating: "Do
not make changes immediately." So I gave myself the gift of time to care
for my body, mind, and soul.

The breakthrough happened by coincidence while reading Louise
Hay's book, You Can Heal Your Life, as she discussed resistance to change.
As I read it, I visualized an imaginary bridge and crossed it to the next
island. It just happened as simply as that. My fear of failure disappeared.
I no longer viewed leaving my job as a failure. I was good enough just for

being myself. I felt empowered to do something about a work situation that had troubled me for a year. Finally, the time had come for change. I trusted that God had a better plan for me. I was hopeful. I trusted that good things would come with ease.

As I left my job, I was worried I would have too much time and not know what to do with it. I had no idea how to live life without thinking about work twenty-four /seven. That was my first real vacation in nineteen years. I developed a bucket list. I travelled, visiting my parents in Lebanon, my brother Malek in Seattle, and my friend, Angele, in Kentucky. I took care of my wellbeing, living a slower pace and putting healthy eating first. I was able to switch off and not worry. I read a lot of books. I did simple activities that filled my happiness tank and calmed my nervous system.

I was eager to learn new modalities in the field of holistic healing. I had heard of Qigong, a Chinese century old system of body postures, breathing and meditation practiced for cultivating energy. I googled Qigong and found a class in a nearby park in Seattle two mornings a week. I loved the calmness and vitality that I gained during the practice.

While in Seattle, I was also eager to discover the power of touch in balancing energy. I found a course on Healing Touch, an energy therapy that utilizes the hands to achieve physical, emotional, mental and spiritual health. During the four days of the workshop, we learnt about the technique and practiced on each other. We would scan each other's bodies, easing blockages and calming emotions. It worked. I was in love with all things alternative. Many people ask me which modality they should begin with? The simple answer is any modality. Once you are ready to explore energy medicine, you will come across someone who knows one. Start with the one that comes to you.

I did not invest too much time searching for a job. I had applied for two jobs as I was leaving my previous company and one materialized within three months. Thanks to my ex-boss Amelle, it turned out to be the least stressful hiring process I had experienced so far. She created a personalized meditation to support me ahead of my interviews. I would close my eyes and visualize my importance in the eyes of God. I would feel wanted and desired. I would anchor myself in my competence and ability to attract good opportunities. I would imagine a smooth interview where communication was flowing and all parties were having fun. It worked!

I went back to work after a three-month break. I was excited to earn a salary again. The job was smaller than my previous role. That was ideal, as I wanted to have a better work life balance. I promised myself that it would be my last corporate job before I made a bigger shift. Things did not turn out the way I expected. There was lots of screaming at the office. I tried not to take it personally, but in reality I did not like the company culture, and was suppressing myself to survive. I was suffering, I felt I was about to break open at any moment and go back to overeating.

I lasted in this job for five months. I fondly remember the moment I spoke up and said: *No More*! For the first time in my life, someone was standing up for me. That someone happened to be me. In hindsight, here I was at the age of forty-one having my first fuck you moment! The teenager in me was on fire. My inner child was victorious. Time had arrived for Rouba to say *enough*. I believe God sent me a scarecrow to give me the courage to leave corporate life. I am thankful for this gift.

As I was scrolling Linked In after my resignation, an article on the "encore career" phenomenon popped up. It discussed a trend among early fifty-year old corporate leaders quitting their careers for something more meaningful. The author was commenting that this trend was now being followed by younger executives in their late thirties and early forties. I had never heard of this before. *Thank you author, that was me, message received.*

After a twenty-year career, I was ready to redirect my life. I was aware that the perks of the corporate world had kept me in a golden cage. I wondered whether on my deathbed, I would remember my achievements of helping the company stock increase in value, my salary raises, awards and bonuses. I had been invested in my work, too busy proving to myself that I mattered. I was yearning for a personal legacy and was now ready to build the next half of my life.

I wasn't sure whether to stay in Dubai or leave. I had a major tile workover done in my living room a few days after my resignation. As I cleared the area, I asked myself: *what if I were packing my belongings to leave this apartment permanently? Am I ready to move out?* My intuition said *yes*. A few days earlier, I had received a call from the developer of my Lebanese apartment informing me that it would be ready in about two months. I remembered the call and realized I could ship my furniture to Beirut.

While I visualized my home belongings in a ship crossing the Arabian Gulf, my soul told me: *follow.*

I listened, since I had learned to trust my intuition as a result of all of the effort I had put into building my self-confidence. It's funny how my mind had zero say in this process. I did not have to think. My intuition just decided. Summer was about to start in Dubai and I could not envision spending an eighth summer in the desert. I was keen on finding love. Ironically, eight years ago, I had moved to Dubai with the hope of meeting a significant other. I was now leaving with the same longing for love. I said goodbye to my friends, packed my belongings and returned to Lebanon.

So began my adventure into the unknown. I did not have a set plan. My intention was to take a year off. I had a growing passion for working with people in the wellness field. I was eager to let this passion grow. I enrolled in a few courses abroad and intended to enjoy Lebanon in between. I missed my parents and was looking forward to some quality time together. I arrived to Tripoli, my parent's hometown, and moved in with them. My old bedroom was now my new home base.

I step out

I step out

I step out

I step out

I step out

I step out

I step out

I step out

I step out

I step out

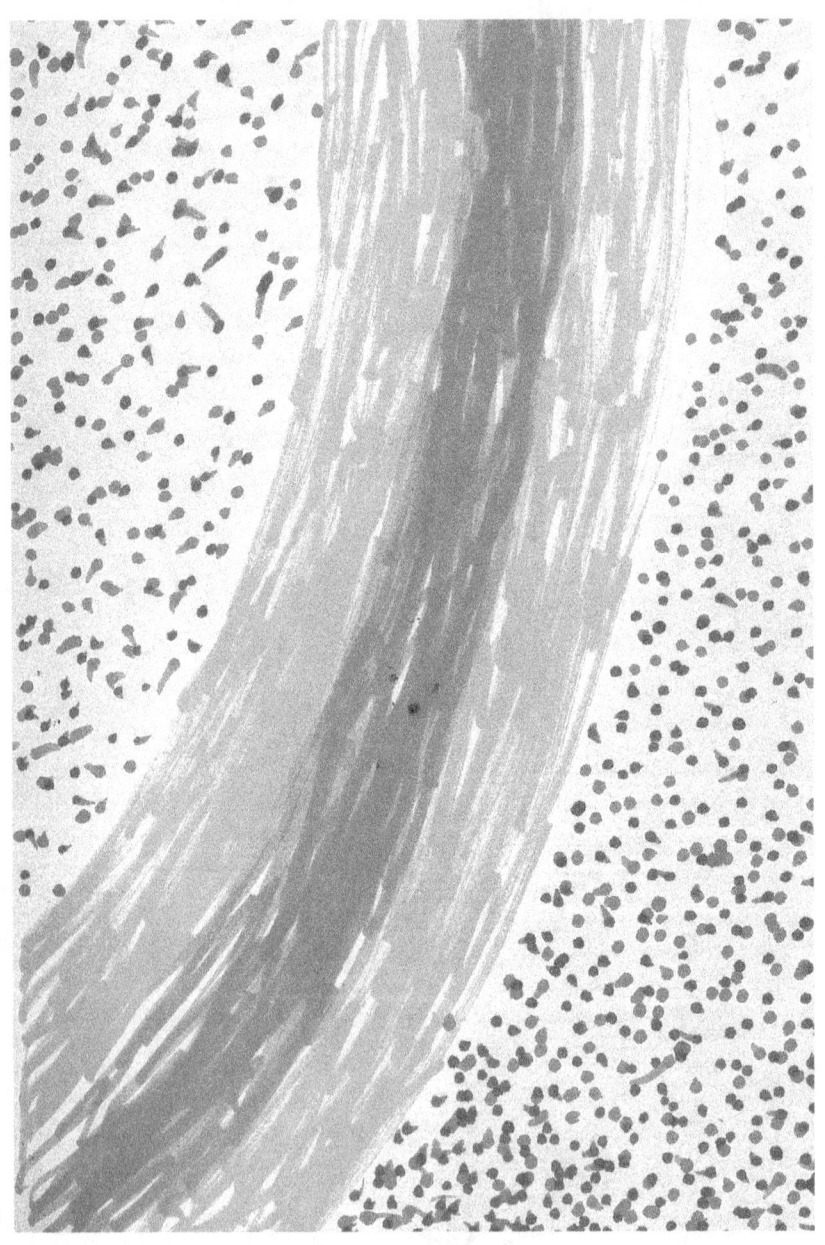

Life is a river

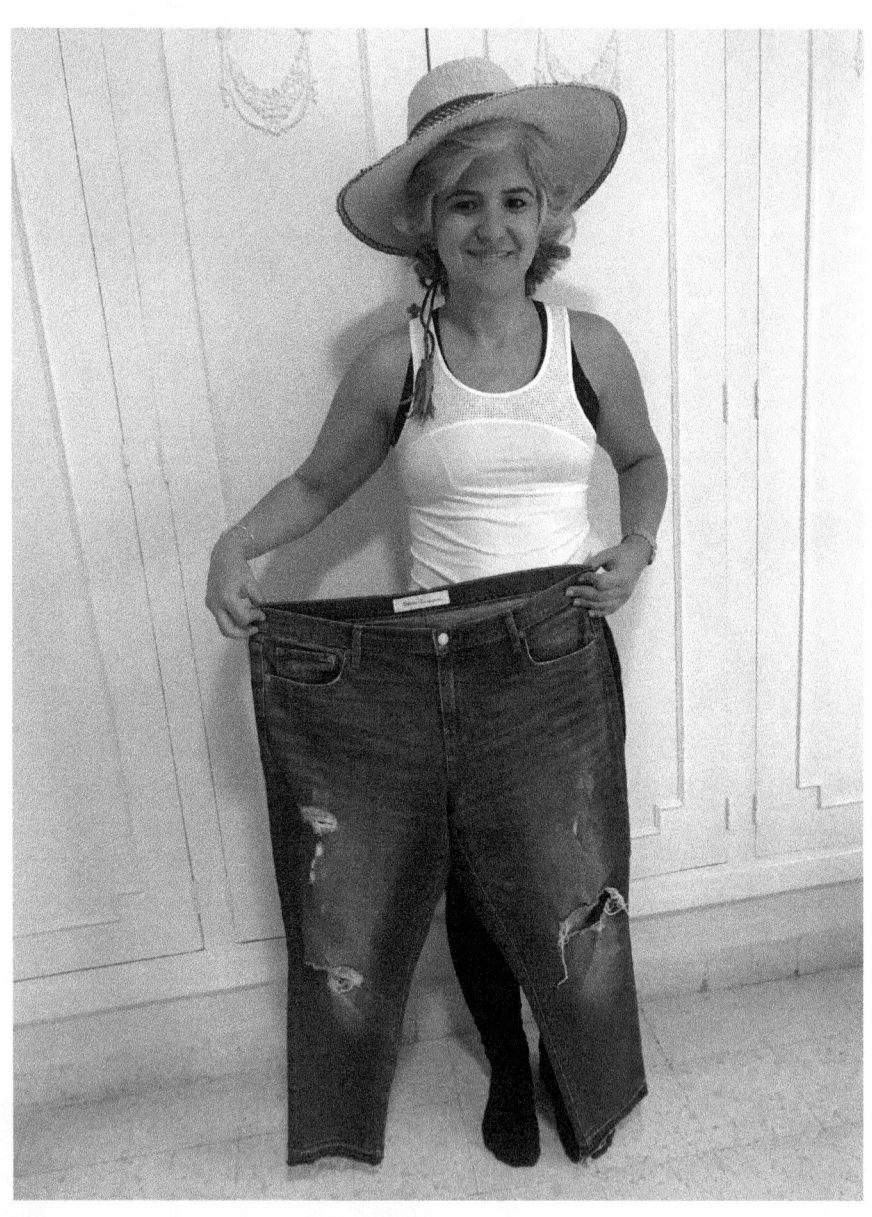

Eighteen months into food addiction recovery

CHAPTER 6

LIVING THIN

■

Life is a journey, not a destination.

- Ralph Waldo Emerson

Once the euphoria of reaching my target weight had settled, I came to the realization that what I had been doing for eighteen months was not over yet, and that my journey was ongoing. The target weight is not the destination. Becoming thin is not the destination. Weight release is just the beginning. While I had somehow completed my physical transformation, other parts of my being were beginning to grasp how to find fullness outside of food. Maintaining the weight was the continuation of this new beginning. I wished I could just freeze my body and remain thin. Unfortunately, that was not possible.

I needed to invest myself further into my emotional and spiritual transformation. I struggled with this lifetime commitment of a recovering food addict who needs to follow a certain life protocol to remain thin. *How could I sustain this path of loving kindness?* I had stopped resorting to 'feel good interventions' that brought instant temporary relief, and instead was committing to a journey of self-care.

In those days when my emptiness was biting, I would switch into emergency status and mobilize all my resources to care for myself. Whenever food thoughts increase and overeating slips begin, I would realize that it is now time for a calming down intervention. I would cancel social activities, retreat to my cave and do everything at my pace. I would get to a beautiful middle where my energy rises, my stomach is calm, my body is thankful and my mind is at peace. This middle would soon veer into the opposite direction. Boredom would slowly build up and make me restless, increasing food thoughts, and temptations. That is when I know it's time for me to reach out and have a social intervention. My energy would rise, calling my spirit alive, placing me in the middle again. Over-socializing would wreak havoc with my rhythm, so within days, I would find myself slipping back into the danger zone.

While I realized that I needed this balance of the social versus the self, I was constantly irritated by the ups and downs. The Muslim culture has an adage that *'one should do everything in moderation.'* If only I could press pause on this middle ground where my healthy eating is an effortless flow. Osho explains:

> To be exactly in the middle means to be dead... To be in the middle is not a static state, it is a dynamic phenomena... You cannot be in the middle, you move from right to left and left to right, this is the only way to remain in the middle.

The middle is indeed a dynamic place and that was exactly what I was struggling with. While my mind loved static things, I came to realize that self-care is not a rigid mental construct but rather a fluid process of gently tending to my evolving needs. While I continued to struggle with the dynamic nature of my equilibrium, I was fluidly learning how to bring my body, emotions, and soul to a center of ease.

I missed those days where I resorted to the 'unhealthy feel good interventions' that would tranquilize me immediately. On the bright side, I had found a workable solution to my overeating struggles. I was no longer a food slave, subject to incessant urges. This new way of eating was keeping my body balanced. I wondered how I was going to gather the strength to comply to the program all my life? Dara, my food addiction recovery counselor, kept repeating: "focus on the right now." *After all, what is the alternative? Going back to compulsive eating? No!*

I was increasingly aware of an aching hole inside my soul, a deep emptiness that cried hunger many times. In the past, I resorted to food, material acquisitions, and status to fill this hole. I now needed to go beyond the emptiness and continue searching for fullness outside of food. As I was leaving Dubai, my food addiction counselor recommended a program in Florida to help me become a counselor.

Phil Werdell is one of the biggest authorities on food addiction with twenty-five years of experience in its treatment and recovery. I had heard of him so much, and I was looking forward to becoming his student. After all, I was passionate about food addiction and its approach to overeating. I was eager to introduce this program to Lebanon as a whole, and my entourage in particular. Most importantly, I wanted to help myself first, now that I would no longer have a supporting community around me. I spent three weeks in Florida with Phil, other experts, and fellow recovering food addicts.

During the program, I experienced a constant need to drink water. Thanks to Phil, I got to understand that this was an indirect way to swallow my emotions. He helped me connect to my fear and anger, which I had been suppressing since childhood, and they came out in full force. I was shocked. I just did not realize how much was bottled up inside of me. I felt relieved yet odd, as though letting go was shameful, or unacceptable even.

I left Florida with a greater curiosity about the world of addiction, specifically food addiction. Thanks to Phil, I now had a long list of books to read while I reflected upon my journey as a recovering food addict and counselor.

■

THE IN-BETWEEN

Goodbye familiar past!
Welcome unknown future!
Bye bye order,
Hello chaos.
Wow I am a free bird!
Hmmm, I am disoriented.
Yay! I am feeling such aliveness.
Ohhh! I am so terrified!
Will I fly?
Will I fall?
I allow life to unfold in the in-between.
Today is not the past, nor the future
It is the magical process, where I become.

■

CHAPTER 7

FEELING PAIN

■

It doesn't interest me what planets are squaring your moon. I want to know if you have touched the center of your own sorrow. If you have been opened by life's betrayals or have become shriveled and closed from fear of further pain.

- Oriah Mountain Dreamer

As I left the certainty of my predictable life, my therapist recommended a retreat that would help me find direction in my transition. The Path of Love calendar showed an offering in Greece in June. I had always dreamt of visiting the Greek Islands in late spring. I signed up without hesitation and came to the Osho Afroz Meditation Center intending to spend ten days. I ended up spending the whole summer.

The Greek countryside had a lot to offer. The center was nestled in an orchard, about ten minutes by car from the beach. That was the kind of setting I needed to recharge after being in the desert for seven years. I was struggling with low energy and a lot of physical pain. I participated in many week-long workshops in support of my inner transformation. In between, my days were filled with time in nature, meditation, dance, reading, journaling, rest, and socializing. I would often go down to the village or the beach.

Through meditation, I went inwards. *"Everything in the universe is within you"* Rumi says. I had been running away from my darkness all my life. I had left jobs and places because I felt imprisoned and suffocated. Now was the time for greater internal awareness, knowledge, and development. I would breathe and connect to my expanding and collapsing chest. I would then feel my heartbeat. Light as a butterfly, I would float in and

and land on each cell of my body and feel its inner state. Rather than judging whether it's tense or relaxed and rushing to fix it, I would practice presence. I would repeat to myself: *I am here, right now, together forever. I love you, we are one.* I sometimes got restless during meditation. I wanted to escape from this practice, since I would find myself distracted, resisting this inward journey. Sometimes, I would fall asleep or space out.

I came to Greece with the intention of becoming strong again. I hated this fragility inside of me. While I was comfortable with energies of strength and control, I disliked being weak, exposed and naked. Whenever faced with negative emotions, I would rise above them and try to recycle them into positive ones. My Path of Love facilitator Satyarti Peloquin invited me to feel the pain. He explained: "You can't feel pleasure and joy if you do not feel pain." I had grown up believing that pain was a weakness. I was never in pain for years, thanks to food. After my bicycle accident, pain just splashed in my face and somehow did not want to go. I just wanted to wipe it out by simply pressing delete.

I learnt to sit with pain. While meditating, I would practice holding space for myself by embracing my emotional storm with a blanket of caring. I would tell myself: *I see you, I hear your suffering, I am not judging you. I am present and staying with you.* I felt very much like an adult Rouba, the mamma, holding the hand of the suffering little Rouba. When I began, I could barely stand the pain. With time, I came to realize that pain dissolves into thin air, when we practice a loving presence and accept ourselves, just the way we are, without any sense of urgency to fix anything. The storm passes and the sun rises.

I was filled with terror. I could not comprehend where all this fear had been stored all those years. I was a courageous woman and never afraid. I had now been broken open. I had a deep conviction that when I am in trouble, no one will be there for me. My fear was real. My fear was old, ingrained, and difficult to overcome.

To help deal with my fear, I did fifteen days of childhood and sexual deconditioning work that took me back to some unpleasant chapters. I was sexually abused by successive female house helpers until about the age of 10. Till today, I do not have a clear recollection of the events, as I had suppressed them. I don't understand how and when it started and why it continued. I have memory fragments from two separate incidents with two different abusers. While I don't recall their faces nor their names, I do remember what the rooms looked like; that at least was safe to remember. I never discussed those abuses with anyone during my childhood. I was afraid I would be punished. Frankly, I didn't feel anybody cared about me.

I had never shared them with anyone until they surfaced during a Thetahealing session a year earlier. The fellow student was trying to dig deeper into the root cause of my lack of trust. Then suddenly, I understood: *I can't trust people because when bad things happened to me, the closest ones were not there.* I blurted out the sexual abuse and began crying. I wanted to hide underneath the table, as I felt that my skin was burning and melting. Thankfully the teacher came to our rescue and calmed me down through positive downloads that *I am safe, I know how and when to be safe and that I am actually safe right now, protected and supported.* I was able to close this chapter until it came up in Greece a year later.

I exploded in rage. *Why me? Why was I the victim of successive abusers? Was it my fault? Where were my parents? Why hadn't they protected me?* I was angry at myself for having allowed this abuse. I was angry at my parents for never being there for me. I felt shame boiling in my blood and bones. I cried and screamed. Each vein in my head was on the verge of bursting out with the suppressed abuse that I feared would wipe me out.

Although this shame had been in my system for more than thirty years, I had contained it in a deep, locked drawer. The abuse did haunt me multiple times a week, or sometimes on a daily basis. The memory was like a virus: attacking my blood and spreading poison. Yet, I was able to ignore it and move on believing that all was under control. Thanks to Gabor Mate and his many books on addiction, I came to understand later on that addicts develop a dullness in feeling as a survival mechanism to unbearable pain. Now I knew where this emptiness came from, and how food supported it. I became intensely sick after this outburst in Greece; I was lethargic and could barely move for weeks. Thankfully I was in a meditation center, surrounded by nature, a loving community, a lot of supporting activities, and a variety of interactions.

In one of the workshops, I remembered the feelings I experienced as a baby. I felt unwelcome when I was born. I felt that my arrival did not matter. I was shocked by this realization, and developed a throat infection for a week. In some ways, I felt I was betraying my parents. I trusted my intuition though, and was able to discern that my feeling was authentic. It made sense as I had easily felt rejected throughout my life. I was always super sensitive to how welcoming or hurtful people were. Many times, I would leave or shut down because I felt rejected.

I discussed it with my sister Rania. She was in Lebanon for the summer and was looking for a temporary place to live in. While visiting apartments, she came across two posters displaying front pages of newspapers from 1976, my birth year. Those newspapers dated a month before and after I was born. They detailed the daily events of the Lebanese civil war. I now had a starting point for a discussion with my mother.

Mom's recollection of the days preceding and following my birth were quite unpleasant. It was wartime. Unknowingly to all of us, the baby in me had sensed their distress and interpreted their distraction as rejection. It's funny how early life events shape us and create limiting beliefs that we sustain through adulthood. Those feelings contaminated my life and infected me with shame. I never expressed them and never realized they were the result of war trauma. Now I know better. Anytime I feel unwelcome, I re-anchor myself in my parents' and friends' love.

I have benefited a lot from sitting with my pain and acknowledging it. Considering it from an external perspective was scary at first. I had avoided pain all my life for fear of losing control. I now knew that pain was liberating me. I became more creative. I began drawing and writing poetry. I began to feel joy and pleasure, which had never been the case before. Mostly, feeling pain allowed me to become whole just like Jalaja Bonheim explains it:

> We achieve true wholeness only by embracing our fragility and sometimes, our brokenness. Wholeness is a natural radiance of Love, and Love demands that we allow the destruction of our old self for the sake of the new.

As in any birth, life only comes after a labor of pain.

I cry
my pain
tears in my eyes
itchy throat
tingling ears
pain in my
    shoulders
heaviness in my
heart
I am lost I am
tired I want to
Ride
A ah aah aah

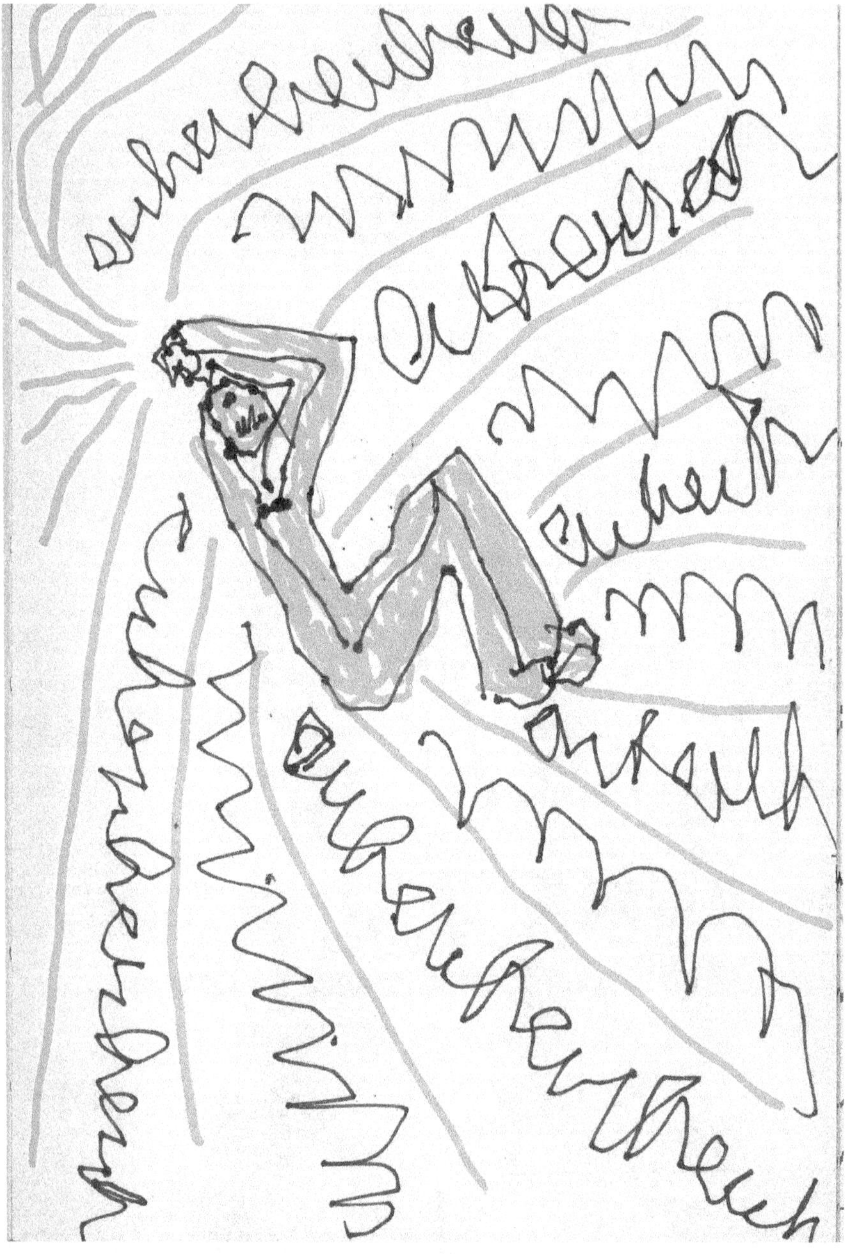

I am afraid
no one loves me
I am alone
See me I am
here
See me
See me
I am afraid

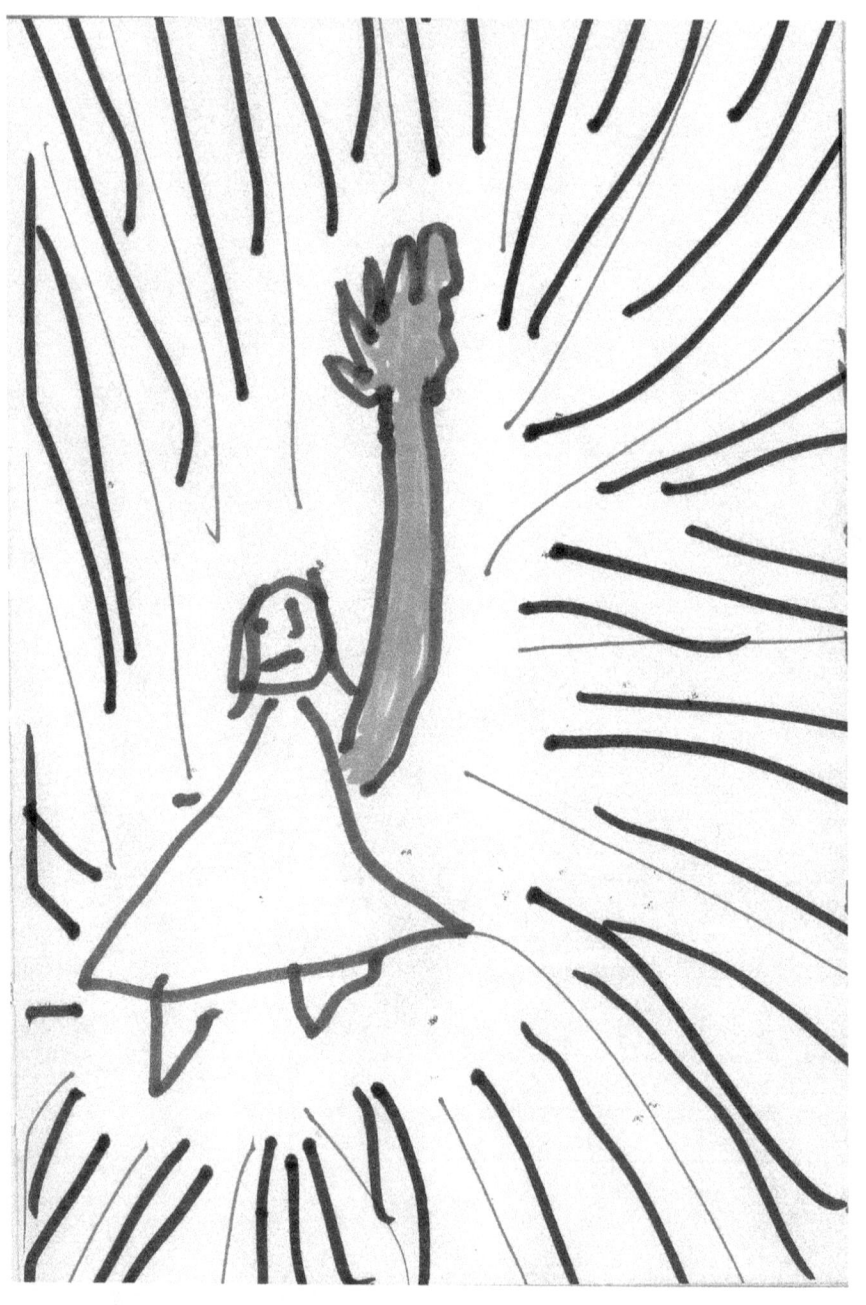

CHAPTER 8

BECOMING NOBODY

■

You spent the first half of your life becoming somebody. Now you can work on becoming nobody, which is really somebody. For when you become nobody, there is no tension, no pretense, no one trying to be anyone or anything. The natural state of the mind shines through unobstructed and the natural state of the mind is pure love.

Ram Das

Who am I? As a young girl, I wanted to be an independent woman, fleeing society's expectation of my role as a wife and a mother. I poured my energy into becoming an accomplished woman. I felt like a jockey constantly hitting a running horse with a stick. My superwoman identity was a reaction to the defect I perceived inside of me. My mom's criticism of my dad made me feel inherently flawed. I rejected and suppressed many parts of me in order to earn my family's and society's respect and admiration. There was no room for mistakes or play. I stood tall and strong, becoming successful and reliable. All aspects of my life were under tight control in service to my perfectionist identity. Perhaps this was driven from my new knowledge of feminism that I superimposed on the way I was raised, where the woman, mother, daughter was under the rule of the father, husband, or brother.

At forty, the status of an independent woman did not give my life the meaning I wanted. I rebelled against the fat, overworked, unmarried, workaholic, cash machine and began a journey of detaching myself from her. There was no need to force myself to do this, so that others would not perceive me this way or that way. I was now able to remove my mask, and see my naked self without titles, labels or fixed identities. I felt liberated from the pressure to conform to my internalized expectations of what I was supposed to be. Jeff Foster says it beautifully:

> Destroy who you were, become all that you are. I'll tell
> you what awakening is: the disappearance of your interest
> in maintaining a consistent image of "Me."

I became gentle. I looked into the eyes of this beautifully imperfect woman and embraced her essence. I gave her permission to just be. I gave her permission to cry. I melted in this kindness. I was in no hurry to become yet. My attention shifted from doing to being. I had all the time in the world to rest and play. I listened to my intuition and allowed my heart to guide my actions. I felt reborn. I could feel a new energy rising in me.

I had many moments of doubt. At times, I could not recognize the person I was becoming. I would feel disoriented. I refused to go back to my old identity, yet I felt lost. Thankfully, I was in Greece surrounded by fellow travelers who had also lost their direction in the journey of life. Osho Afroz meditation center offered daily evening meetings outdoors under a beautiful oak tree. We would begin the session by dancing for twenty minutes and then listening to a discourse by Osho. I was never fully focused, but somehow his words would suddenly prick my attention:

> You are not accidental. Existence needs you. Without you
> something will be missing in existence and nobody can
> replace it. That's what gives you dignity, that the whole
> existence will miss you. The stars and sun and moon, the
> trees and birds and earth – everything in the universe
> will feel a small place is vacant which cannot be filled by
> anybody but you.

Thank you Osho, *yes I mattered. Existence would not be the same without me. I am here for a reason. The reason is not that important. What matters is my presence. There is no need to justify my presence. I am simply here, just here.*

I felt homeless. Many nights, my soul would roam through Dubai.

I longed for the comfort and safety of the home that I had left. As I meditated, I would imagine a pin going deep into the earth underneath me: I would remind myself that *my home is inside of me, my home is being present right here and right now.*

As I returned to society, people challenged me. Many wanted to understand what was happening, and what my plans were. In my moments of doubt, I would remember Eckhart Tolle:

> Give up defining yourself – to yourself and others. You won't die. And don't be concerned about how others define you. When they define you, they are limiting themselves, so it's their problem. Whenever you interact with people, don't be there primarily as a function or role, but as a field of conscious presence. You can only loose something that you have, but you can't loose something that you are.

All my life, I had gained my self-worth from my accomplishments, now I was ok being myself, a "nobody" in free form. That was freeing, empowering, and relieving. I did not need to earn my space in this universe. I had nothing to prove to anyone, or myself. I existed full stop, thanks to the life inside me. This unapologetic presence was a new and fun feeling.

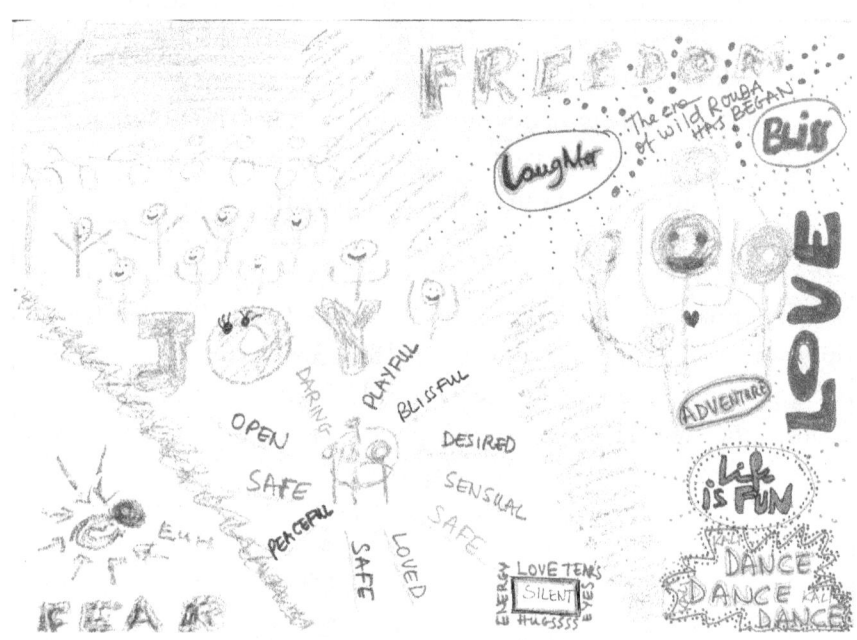

Walking the path of freedom

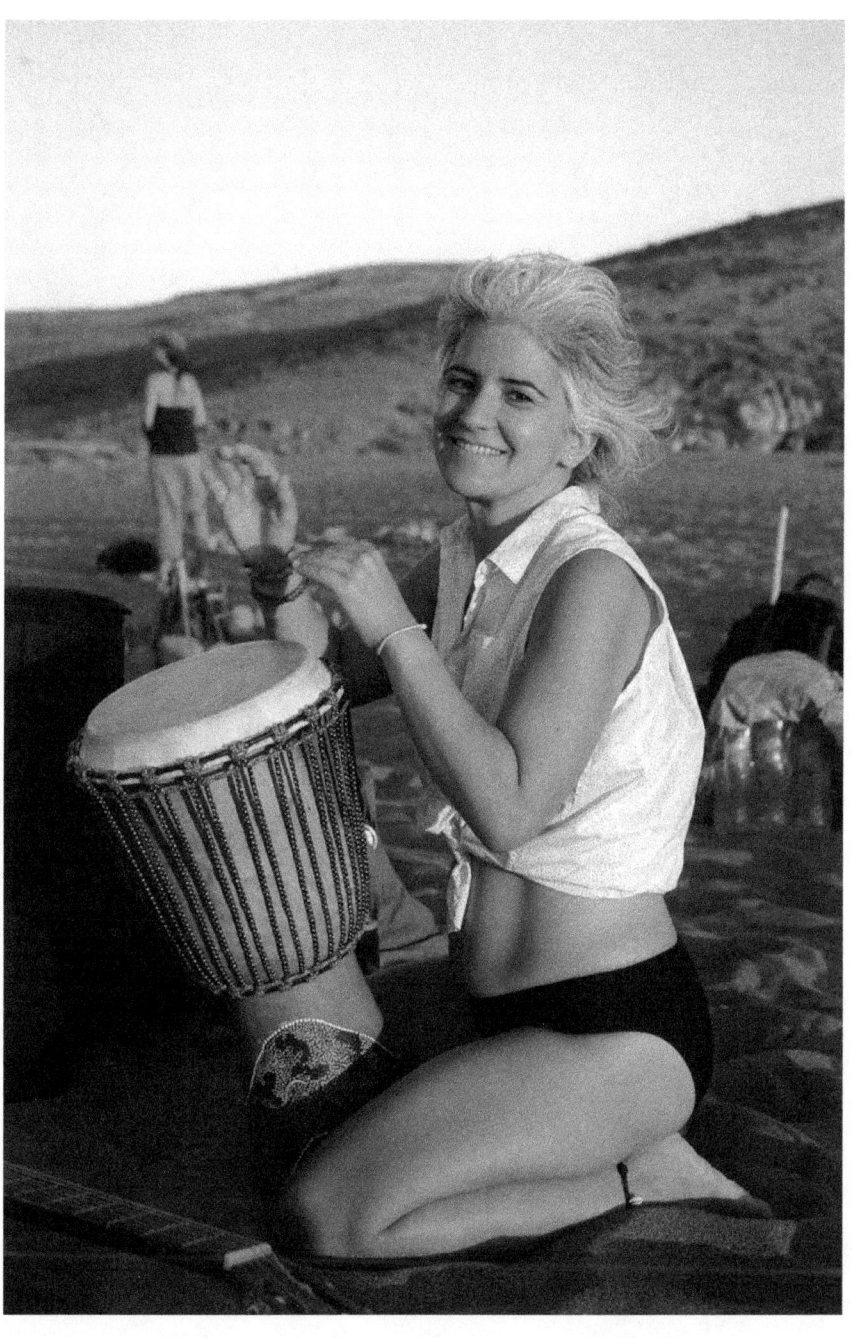

CHAPTER 9

OPENING UP TO LOVE

■

Your task is not to seek for love, but merely to seek and find all the barriers within yourself that you have built against it.

- Rumi

At forty, I felt totally incompetent at attracting love. Male interactions rarely lasted beyond four weeks, except for a seven-month relationship that was a total disaster. I was lonely, unmarried and childless. I was bitter and angry.

While growing up, I never felt deserving of anyone's love. That's quite a painful realization now. My parents' relationship did not inspire me. It felt to me like a prison: somehow they had been condemned to stay together. In our family context and their generation, divorce was not socially conceivable. I did not want to end up like my mother, a housewife married at sixteen, who was wholly dependent on her husband and family. I was terrified of having a husband as disconnected as my father. My sexual abuse did not help. I unconsciously discarded my body and avoided any possibilities for anyone getting close and touching me. Food comforted me. Being fat and ugly was in no way marriage material. After all, I did not trust men. I was too afraid they would hurt me.

I became interested in love in my mid-twenties after most of my friends had gotten married. I felt lonely and the odd one out among my married friends and cousins. I was eager to tick the box. My experience ranged from disappointment to disillusionment. I would open up and allow men in, only to feel overwhelmed. I would become disenchanted within days or a maximum of two weeks, then close myself again for a year or two. Finding love was one of my major motivations to leave Lebanon in my thirties. I did not feel I had a chance here given the seven women to one man ratio. Dubai looked more promising. That was not the case. Men were interested in a more transactional, transient relationship. I struggled. I did psychotherapy and life coaching, I took online courses with love coaches, but nothing seemed to result in a lasting relationship.

I quit corporate life, eager to focus on my personal life. I did not want to be lonely in the second half of my life. I wanted to be loved. I was longing to share my life with a significant other. Thanks to my transformation, I felt better in my own skin, and I had finally given myself permission to fall in love with myself. Yet, I still felt fat inside. My new body in the mirror did not match my inner vision of myself. This began to gradually shift.

While in Greece, I began to see my light in the eyes of others. I no longer felt invisible. I owned my space. God sent me many angels to increase my trust in men. The workshops helped. I was ready to be daring again. I opened up and allowed men in. I also became aware of a protective shield I had built around my heart to protect myself from hurt and rejection. At times, I struggled to lower my defenses, as I was afraid of being totally exposed. Wearing protective armor resulted in my subconsciously keeping others away. I began to softly swing between highly and slightly protective walls.

I fondly remember a letter left to me by Dze with whom I had confided my struggles. She explained that men either came for a reason, a season or a lifetime. I cherish this advice to date, and share it with other friends struggling to find love. Indeed some men entered my life to have me see the goodness in the male gender, or teach me something I needed to learn on my way to building a relationship with a future one. Others came for a season, I needed their support for a time, but afterwards, life had to move on. In the words of Jeff Brown:

> People walk away from love because it is so beautiful that it terrifies them. Sometimes they leave because the connection shines a bright light on their dark places and they are not ready to work them through. Sometimes they run away because they are not developmentally prepared to merge with another... Sometimes they take off because love is not a priority in their lives...Sometimes they end

it because they prefer a relationship that is more practical than conscious, one that does not threaten the ways they organize reality.

Thanks to his wisdom, I stopped taking a man's leaving personally. I realized we were each on our own unique journey. *When a man leaves me, it's not about me, it's about his journey,* and I was finally able to accept that on a deep level. I also became grateful for their contributions to my growth. I started focusing more on my journey rather than the outcome of any interaction.

■

I RECEIVE

I see smiles that make me soften,
Pretty much now and often,
I receive unconditional love,
Embracing me from above.
I receive support and protection
Sensing gratitude and perfection,
I receive grace that makes me flow,
With each touch of abundance I grow.

■

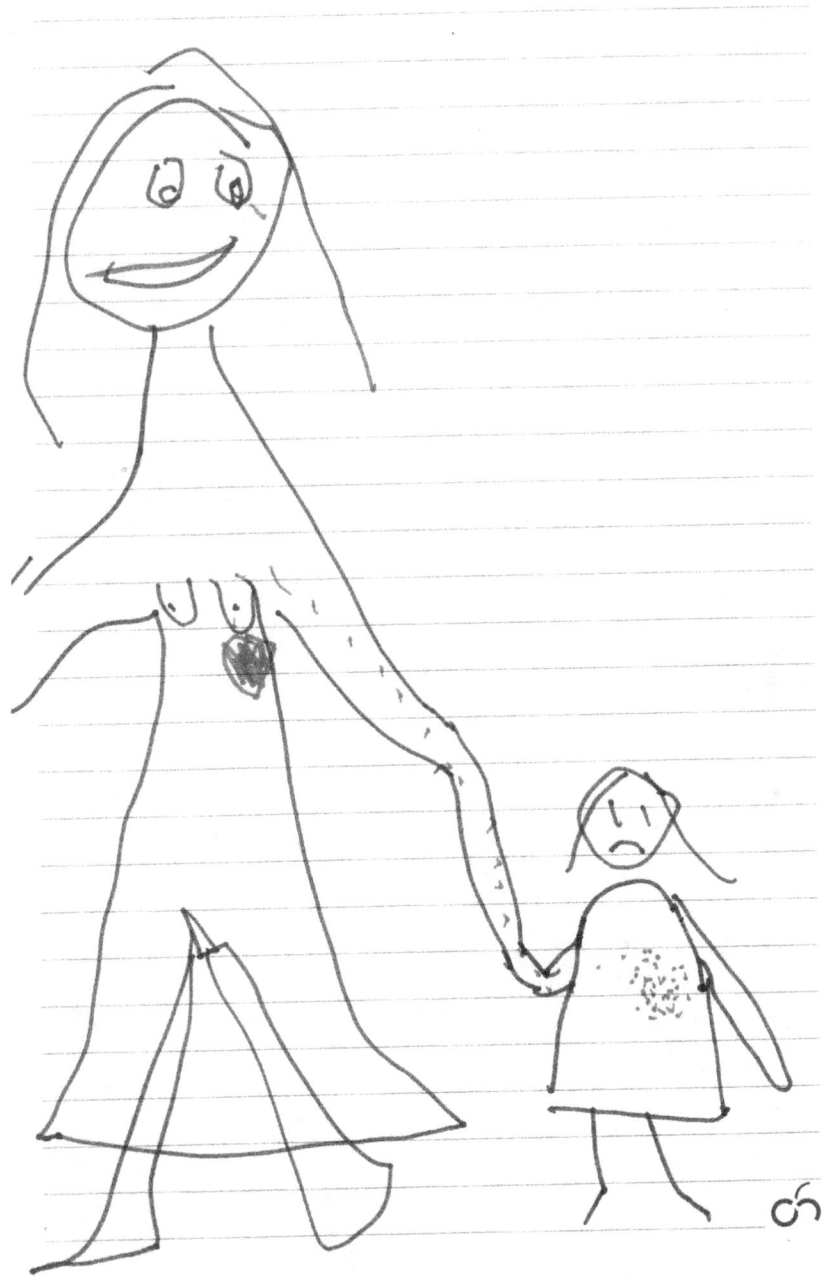

Connecting to my inner child

CHAPTER 10

RESTING IN MY PARENTS' NEST

■

It takes courage to say yes to rest and play in a culture
where exhaustion is seen as a status symbol.

- Brene Brown

As I left Greece, I felt more comfortable with the uncertainty of my transition. I felt ok being confused, as this was unchartered territory. I was open to embracing life as it came, even though sometimes I felt unsettled. I knew it was going to be messy, but that I would be fine. By that point, I was stuck in a roundabout that I kept circling. I was ok with that too. Prior to taking any turn, I now knew that I would need to check whether that direction honored my freedom. I became less attached to the idea of reaching a destination. I wanted to live in the now and enjoy what I was going through.

I was excited about reintegrating into society and digesting all the deep shifts. I returned to Lebanon, to my parent's nest. Our time together was pure nourishment for my soul. As a child, I sometimes felt I was the parent and they were the children. I was happy to go back to my role as a child. I was now filling those love and safety tanks that were left empty during childhood. It felt good. That was exactly what my nervous system needed.

My parents evolved as I evolved. After a health episode, my father expressed interest in following a food addiction recovery meal plan. He lost twenty kilograms (about fort-three pounds) and now looked ten years younger. I was so happy for him. Supporting him in his journey has been challenging yet rewarding. It somehow brought all of our deeply buried issues to the surface. I struggled to communicate with him and thankfully mom was there to ease the relationship. In our eighteen months of living together, I came to accept him as he is, unconditionally. My relationship with my mother continues to deepen. Mom became my guinea pig throughout the holistic modalities I was learning. Our relationship grew stronger, built on love and understanding.

Returning to my parents' nest gave me a sense of normalcy in between my trips. Now that I was home, I could stabilize my body through eating on my schedule and preparing my own food. My body would gradually return to its natural rhythm. I kept a slow pace with a daily routine focused on my wellbeing. I rejoiced in the slow rhythm of my new life. When I lived in a hurry, life felt like rushing on a speeding train. As I began to live slowly, life seemed different. I was present, even embedded, in everything I did.

I enjoyed being back in society. I had fun with mom's friends Zeina and Wafa. We spent time in Tripoli's old town. Together with my friends Marlene and Nehme, we would often go hiking in the mountains. I would regularly do yoga at Bassem's HOM studio. I also slowly reconnected with my friends. I enjoyed spending time with them after being away for so long. Being in society helped me make sense of everything and integrate all those transformations into my new self.

While I made sure to return to Lebanon in between my trips, I could not manage to stay more than three weeks. My apartment in Beirut was far from being ready. Somehow the universe wanted me to travel more. My friend Rana would jokingly warn me that she's about to confiscate my passport. I was enjoying this soul-searching kind of travel and wanted more and more of this inner and outer exploration.

Together with my parents, we travelled to Ghana. I am a fourth generation Ghanaian of Lebanese decent. I grew up in Accra until the age of fifteen. Two of my siblings live there along with most members of my mom's family. I was curious to be back after all the childhood deconditioning work I had done over the summer. Negative emotions would usually re-surface whenever I visited. *How different was this time going to be?*

My three weeks in Ghana were a time of celebration. My sister Rania was curating her third art exhibition, and together as a family, we all wanted to be there for her. As a child, I always felt awkward about celebrations. I did not know how to relax and have a good time. I was always on alert, on the lookout, for any imminent danger. This time, I was breathing and opening myself up to the joy that surrounded me, embracing it wholeheartedly. I received everyone's love with an open heart and went with the flow of all celebrations. I felt alive. I felt light and enjoyed being my new self. It felt good. It felt natural.

Ghana felt different this time around. I made sure to keep a slow routine with daily self-care in the form of reading, meditating, dancing and cooking. By then, I had become an inspiration to many. Everyone was eager to learn about the secret recipe of my wellbeing. I did not have to say anything. My wellbeing expressed itself effortlessly. It is funny how when we don't feel the need to prove ourselves, we shine and everyone notices.

CHAPTER 11

ACCEPTING MYSELF

■

You don't need to be accepted by others. You need to accept yourself.

- Thich Nhat Hanh

Six months after leaving Dubai, I came back for a visit. My pretext was a course that joined two of my interests: Thetahealing and addiction. I was also eager to experience the city that used to be my home following all of my personal transformations. I also missed my friends, whom I had not enjoyed as much as I should have when I was there in the first place.

Unknowingly, I was about to make a big discovery. During the workshop, I found out that I was a highly sensitive person. I love these 'aha moments' when a missing piece of the puzzle illuminates a new corridor of awareness. I have always been particularly sensitive to crowds and excessive noise. While others may enjoy the vibrant energy of busy places, I would easily become unsettled. I never understood why. I felt odd about it throughout my life, and I would sometimes pressure myself to cope, only to be further unsettled for days. I suffered as a child, as my eagerness to shut down and sleep was an annoyance to my cousins during sleepovers. They would try to scare, tickle, or pillow fight me into waking up.

As I researched and read books about being highly sensitive, I stopped forcing myself to cope with crowds and excessive noises and began identifying the signs early on about my need to retreat into a quiet place. Caring for myself after a sensory hangover meant spending time in nature, going to bed early, and having quiet days. While I had intuitively done all of those interventions in the past, they came as a last resort, and were accompanied by a sense of guilt for being anti-social.

My high sensitivity had been a source of shame until I was able to place my finger on it. I was now able to accept myself the way I was. I did not need to apologize for who I was. I now felt that missing out on some events was what was best for me, and that I should just do what my body needs. For many years, I had forcefully exposed my body to too much turbulence. I was now a friend to my body. I listened to what it communicated, responded with love, care, and a deep understanding of its requirements. My body and I were finally at peace.

I loved who I was becoming. It broke my heart that I had always strived to be accepted by others, while denying myself any weakness. Accepting myself now felt so good. It brought tears to my eyes. At last, I was allowing myself to be seen for my true, original, imperfect form unapologetically. While I cherished my strengths, I was now unconditionally accepting of my limitations. That was new and freeing on its own.

My fear popped up again during the workshop. The facilitator and my student buddy Dalia created affirmations to help me anchor myself in my safety: *I know how to speak up when I am in trouble. I know how to shout out for help, when necessary. I am seen, and I am worthy of attention and support. I can visualize myself being rescued.* I still use this framework today whenever I feel insecure. It is reassuring to have it to fall back on when I feel uncertain.

I enjoyed my Dubai visit. I stayed at the home of my ex-colleague Sharmeen, and I was able to catch up with many friends. I was amazed by how much six months had transformed me. I was enjoying my journey and was excited about what life had in store for me.

■

POSSIBILITY

I flow effortlessly,
Bringing grace to my space.
I fly high in the sky,
In this infinity I only see possibility.
This moment is the moment
I am, just, as I am

■

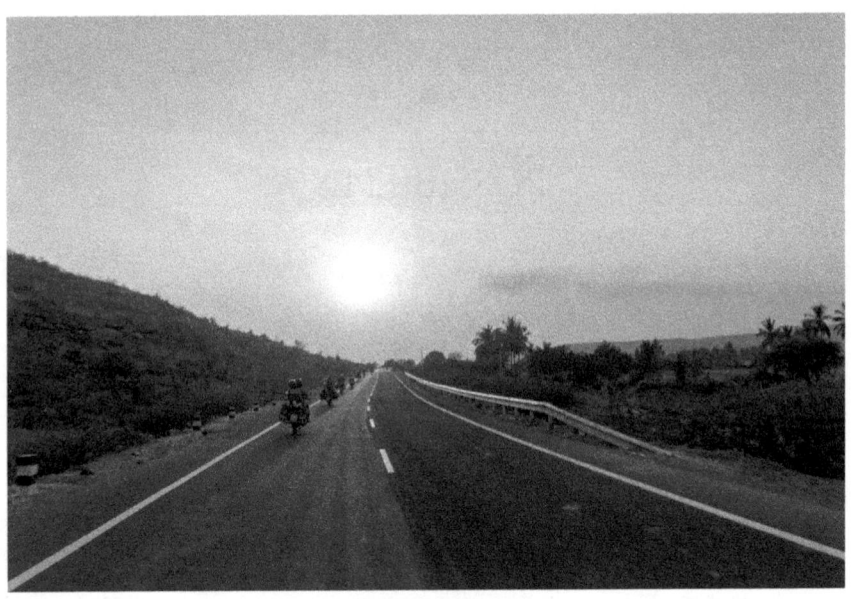

On the roads of India

CHAPTER 12

TRAVELING THROUGH INDIA

∎

Twenty years from now you will be more disappointed by the things that you didn't do than by the ones you did do. So throw off the bowlines. Sail away from the safe harbor. Catch the trade winds in your sails. Explore. Dream. Discover.

- Mark Twain

I was not yet ready to settle in Lebanon. After all, my apartment was not completed yet. I wanted to leave the comfort of my protective walls and go on an adventure of sorts. My friend from Greece, Kristen, got me excited about a motorcycle trip across India. I had heard so much about this great nation of spirituality. This motorcycle trip sounded wild. I did not know how to ride a bike. I contacted the organizer and found out I could join as a passenger. So here I was surrendering myself to angel drivers and trusting the universe to keep me safe. While Kristen changed her mind, I went ahead and signed up with the group, Enfield is Prayer.

The trip began in Siliguri in West Bengal not far away from Nepal and Bangladesh. The city had one long main street with smaller dirt roads. It reminded me of my childhood days in Ghana. I met the rest of the biking group, and together we spent two days getting to know each other while familiarizing ourselves with the motorcycle.

I had initially signed up for one trip of two weeks, and ended up spending a total of 10 weeks in India doing three motorbike trips and resting in between. There was an interesting mix of nationalities: a few Americans, a few Greeks, a Korean, a few Germans, an Indian, a Bulgarian, a few Mexicans, a Swede, a few Dutch and myself, the only Lebanese. I had crossed paths with some of them in Greece. We were all from the Osho world, spiritual nomads in this universe, on a journey of inner and outer exploration. Ours was a small world where birds of a feather flock together.

While I did not drive, I loved being on a motorbike. I was my own version of Marco Polo on an expedition across the Indian subcontinent. We would start riding at sunrise and arrive to our next destination past sunset after having crossed about 200 kilometers. We would drive through highways, small roads, bridges, markets, cities, small towns, villages, forests, agricultural lands, rivers and beaches. The variety was endless. Every day felt like a lifetime.

As a passenger, I spent my time taking in all those sights and sounds, capturing pictures and videos, meditating, and reflecting about humanity and the world. I was blessed by wonderful drivers. I would rotate among Crystal, Pravas, Vikalpo, Chris and Rama. I enjoyed their different driving styles and personalities. We had great conversations too. I was often the designated co-pilot in charge of the route. Being on a motorcycle was a feast for my senses. I felt connected with nature, and the world around me. I felt free.

We made many stops during our driving days. We attended to our personal needs, such as drinking, eating, and relieving our bowels all in nature. We discussed the days ahead and route changes. Sometimes we had to tend to some mechanical or health problems, mostly diarrhea, vomiting and nausea. Our days were filled with surprises.

Everywhere we went, we were met with kindness. The sparkly eyes, open arms and smiles are forever engraved in my heart. On one of our stops, the whole village gathered around us within twenty minutes. I felt like a Martian, the differences in the ways we dressed, talked, and behaved were at odds with those we met. It was surreal. We interacted with many school children, whose innocence and curiosity were refreshing, and I was struck with their easy acceptance of us. My heart warms up as I remember the magic of our encounters.

Everywhere we travelled, I could feel India growing. There were road constructions everywhere. Most road construction workers were women working in their beautiful saris. There was so much color and grace in the midst of all the dust, noise, and the smell of heated tar. I don't think I have ever seen as many trucks in my life: kilometers and kilometers of trucks. I saw lots of buses and motorcycles too, while cars were a rare commodity. I loved the rickshaws, India's fit for purpose transport solutions: a crossover between a motorcycle and a car. Their usage ranged from transporting people, to carrying agricultural produce.

I was impressed by India's management of waste at a local level. India has a caste of waste pickers. They live picking food from waste and somehow sorting the waste and burning what's left. The waste picker ladies looked beautiful in their colorful saris, jewelry and eye make up. Plastic bag use was scarce across India. Instead, everyone used colorful fabric bags. In the city of Pune, I saw outdoor vacuum cleaners for the first time in my life.

Everywhere I went, I saw lactating dogs with puppies. The cycle of life was omnipresent no matter where we went. I saw plenty of cows, kittens, and little monkeys; except for the naughty monkeys, all other animals were peaceful. It made me sad as I contrasted them with the enraged Lebanese dogs. I reflected about our notion of space and property in Lebanon, where people have very defined views about borders. They would abuse dogs for trespassing or kill birds for pooping on their clothes, or remove trees because they are dirtying their cars. In India, all are welcome everywhere, food is shared, together people and animals are part of the cycle of life. Somehow the enraged Lebanese dog is a representation of our enraged disconnected Lebanese society; another one is the crazy drivers replaying the war on our highways.

I loved the contentment and peacefulness of Indians. I remember a visit to a shoemaker. Seated in a meditative position by the sidewalk, he repaired shoes and leather goods all day. His calm and craftsmanship were admirable. He was in total flow with his work. He was at peace with life. I loved this live encounter with surrender, which is in sharp contrast with the restlessness of the Lebanese, whose complaints, anger, and dissatisfaction is loud and burdensome.

We stayed in many towns along our odyssey, spending a day or two in some locations. I was privileged to visit a few pilgrimage sites. Bodhi Gaya is the Buddhist Mecca. It's located on the site of the Bodhi tree where Buddha got enlightened. There, we met pilgrims from all over Asia and the world. We visited Varanasi, the Hindu equivalent of Jerusalem and Rome. The city has been continuously inhabited for thirteen thousand years. Hindu pilgrims come to Varanasi to wash away their sins in the sacred waters of the river Ganga, cremate their loved ones, or simply die in the hope of reaching Nirvana and being liberated from the cycle of rebirth and reincarnation. As one of the oldest continuously inhabited cities, Varanasi has many alleyways and a vibrant culture. I struggled around this energy of death, as a part of me was dying too. I believe that dying in this city is a journey of rebirth rather than simply death. Somehow many of us got a stomach bug after such a long trip in the sun and constant exposure to nature. We were tired from days of riding and this was a good opportunity to rest and relax before we hit the road again.

We visited a few Unesco heritage sites, like the Khajurahu's erotic temples that seemed to possess magical energy. Their fine sculptures and Kama Sutra depictions are among the most beautiful I have ever seen. I enjoyed being lost in the alleys of Badami, dreaming of how this place would have looked like, centuries ago, at the pinnacle of that civilization. I would not have minded being forgotten there by the group in the magnificence of this site. Its red rocks had such a strong energy.

We visited towns by the river. Orchha was the glorious capital of the Bundelkhand kingdom. There are many palaces that overlook the Betwa River, which splits into multiple channels. As the Arabic saying goes, this place extended my life thanks to just meditating and singing by its river. It had the feel of One Thousand and One Arabian Nights. Hampi is another magical place with temples and rivers. Thankfully, the weather was warm enough to swim in its blessed water, which helped me feel rested, accepted, and healed. Hampi has magnificent rock formations by the water, which form wonderful pools that only need a painter to honor them properly. I can still hear the water echoing underneath them, the sound of its flow triggering a sense of peace that I felt all over my body.

We passed through many beach towns in Goa and its surrounding states. I mostly enjoyed waking up at sunrise and walking on empty beaches while everyone else was asleep. The wonder and colors that I woke up to gave me back the joy that I had lost in the course of my adult, fast paced life. I can still hear the echoes of Indian spiritual music played by the first shift of workers, setting up the beach house for breakfast.

Coping with the group dynamics took a lot of my energy, especially when the group became larger. Finding common ground among all of us was more difficult, and the logistics more complex. As a highly sensitive person, I struggle with too much talking and socialization, and need time to myself. I also suffer when it gets too disorganized. I struggled to find suitable food options without sugar and flour. Thanks to my friend Lana, all the way in Dubai, I was able to find some workarounds. I stocked up on my food and had back up plans for emergency situations. I refrained from sharing my food, so that I would not run out of what I needed to eat. Thankfully the fruits were amazing. Nothing beats Indian pomegranates and strawberries.

We completed our motorbike pilgrimage in Pune. I was a wreck after being on the road for 4,000 kilometers. I had fallen off the motorcycle on the last day of the ride and was limping. My energy was scattered and I did not want to go back to Lebanon before I had recovered a bit. I stayed at a hotel that was a few minutes walk from the Osho International Meditation Center, and I spent my days hanging out with some friends I had met on my bike journey. I enjoyed being in the company of Chris, Miriam and Anne. We were delighted to be back to civilization, eating food we had missed, getting massages, and just taking things easy.

I also spent a few days at the Osho Center. By then, I was restless and nothing was calming me down. I felt irritated and was constantly fighting with myself. Thankfully, my cousin Rawah was in Bombay, and we would have long phone conversations, which helped me calm down, but I still did not have the energy to visit her.

As I looked back, I had taken this pilgrimage to India in the hope of achieving an inner reconciliation. After almost a year of transition, I was feeling even more lost. I was having an overdose from being an adventurer. *Where am I? Am I in a dream or a nightmare? Where am I heading?* Life felt absurd. I had still not met my loved one. I was full of doubts about everything. I was tired, angry, and sarcastic. I felt that I had once again hit rock bottom.

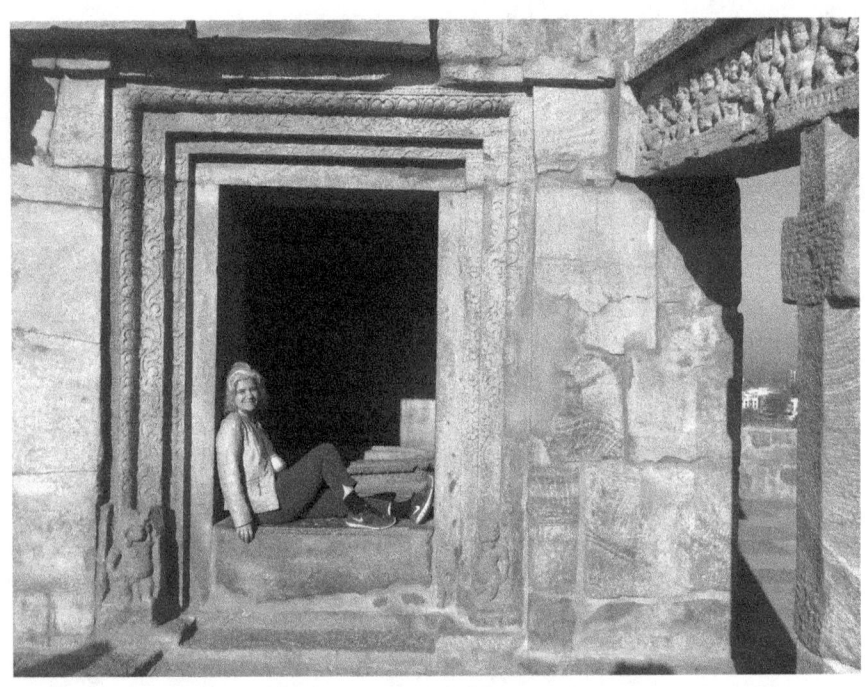

In India as I swing between fullness and emptiness

■

GOD

I feel the warmth of your protection
With certainty and conviction
I feel safe everyday
As you bless my way!

■

Future

{in-between}

Past

BECOMING
"GROWTH"

Future	Becoming	Past
Uncharted waters	Messy	Familiar
unknown	Fear / scary	
Exciting	uncomfortable	Stillness
Exhilirating	tense clumsy	Boring
	raw	Prison
	chaotic	Suffocating
	exploration	
	Freedom	
	Flying & Falling	

CHAPTER 13

FINDING LOVE AFTER DARKNESS

■

Sometimes when you're in a dark place, you think you've been buried, but you've actually been planted.

- Christine Caine

By the end of my India trip, I was back in a dark tunnel, and feeling stuck in quick sand. I hated this limbo land between my past and my future. I still had a lot of pain and weakness in my body. I felt empty, irritated and impatient. While I knew I needed to rest after being on the road for weeks, I felt I had not been able to gather enough energy to achieve my dream.

I went back to Lebanon to my parents' cocoon. I slept and ate healthy for a whole week and did not leave my bedroom. My mom would peak and ask: "Are you going to keep on sleeping?" I would answer "yes" from the depth of my bed. I just needed to be left alone. I lived day-by-day, tending to my body, and listening to what it needed.

Instagram became my spiritual meditation board. On her page "We Are Soul Sparks", Kristin Lohr writes:

Growth happens when we are suspended in midair not knowing if you'll fly or fall. Growth happens in the in-between.

Lohr gave me the strength to keep on choosing the person I was becoming and believing that I was on the right path. Jeff Foster verbalized my deepest emotions of brokenness. I felt shattered into a zillion little pieces and lost in my journey. Somehow he posted every time I needed him and gave me the reassurance that I was ok. After all, I was not becoming crazy. What I was going through was normal in my journey of transformation.

I reached out to my friends from Greece. With them, I could totally be myself and express my darkest feelings. They provided me with a safe space to express my fears. I felt nourished by their container of love. As I rested, I gained strength and began to leave the house and go to yoga classes. It was springtime and hiking was lovely. I enjoyed the company of my mom and her friends, Wafa and Zeina. My friends Marlene and Nehme would often visit too, and together we would have long walks. Every week or so, I would go to Beirut and spend a night at my friend Sarah's. This was a time of nourishment.

I was keen to achieve progress on the man front. I was not in the mood for outings and had plenty of time to converse via social media. I began to experiment with dating application Tinder. I kept my expectations low given my bad experiences in Dubai. As I scrolled through pictures, I avoided men with fake names and those who would not display their face. I stayed away from those showing party or family pictures. For those whom I was matched with, I would wait until they reached out, and then eliminate anyone quickly if they did not fit with my values. I would ask about their marital status and say goodbye to anyone married. I would chat for a few days until I felt comfortable enough to speak. The men I ended up conversing with were mostly in complicated life situations, with no real interest to meet. Tinder afforded them with virtual solace.

As I looked into changing my selection process, I remembered a friend from Dubai who preferred Tinder Gold. I upgraded my membership to access an option where you can see the men who like you. I would scroll through that list slowly and reflect about the energy of their faces and then press yes or no. This Tinder option gave a valuable shortlist. I hit it off with one guy who was living one kilometer away. After a few days of chatting, he proposed to meet. I remember my friend from India, Anne's advice: "never go on a first meeting at night, always choose a morning or an afternoon coffee; meet him there."

After a successful first meeting, we started seeing each other often. He was kind, loving, caring, and would get me a rose every day. He asked me a killer question after three weeks: "Will you invest in my business?" I was offended. Despite all my work in embracing my feminine energy, it pained me that I was still radiating a cash machine identity. I told him it was over. It was a smooth process and he probably went on his next investment conquest. I focused on the positive. He came into my life for a reason. I was now more open to receiving and readier for my next relationship.

Thanks to my girlfriends' encouragement, I went back to Tinder and met Hadi within days. While an instant attraction formed after our first meeting, I was more cautious this time. After all, he lived abroad. I just went with the flow. I needed to travel after a few days, and I was going to be away for a month.

I struggled in the early stages of our relationship. I found myself searching for his flaws and rationalizing why he was not trustworthy. I was constantly anxious and would easily interpret any of his actions as a rejection. Unknowingly, I was sabotaging our relationship out of fear of being hurt. I began reading Amir Levine's book: Attached: the new science of adult attachment and how it can help find and keep love. As I became aware of my patterns, I was able to express my deepest fears of rejection. Hadi is secure in his love relationships. He was patient and would reassure me: "I am not running away." Through his unconditional love, I became less anxious and did not run in the opposite direction.

Long distance relationships are characterized by short bouts of togetherness bliss amid a sea of separation anxiety. At times, this pattern brought out the worst in me. I thought of quitting as I asked myself what was the purpose of having someone who was not around. I wanted to avoid the pain of our separation. Through his maturity and unconditional love, Hadi knew how to calm me down.

Our love continued to grow. We've been together for a year, breaking my record of the longest relationship. At forty-three, I celebrated my first Valentine. I am no longer afraid that this relationship is not going to last. As I was scrolling through my notes, I found an entry on my phone that I had written two years back: "my man is a rock I can lean on. He is consistent and quiet and has acts of service as his language of love." The universe had manifested Hadi.

I do not worry too much about the future of our relationship. After all, there is no destination. As long as today is good, tomorrow does not matter. I surrender to the flow and allow life to direct the steering wheel of the magic of our togetherness.

CHAPTER 14

BECOMING ALIVE

■

Don't ask yourself what the world needs. Ask yourself
what makes you come alive. And then go do that. Because
what the world needs is people who have come alive.

- Howard Thurman

I have suffered from low energy and have hated physical activity since
childhood. I would easily get exhausted while many friends and cousins
had an oversupply of energy. I felt ashamed for being lazy. Food was my
fuel: sugar gave me instant gratification.

My transformative journey began when my body rebelled and crashed
on the bicycle. In my journey of recovery, I wanted to regain the energy
to achieve any dream I wished. I did not have a particular roadmap in
mind to refill my empty tank, so I began experimenting with whatever
came my way and resonated with me. As I look back, I was pretty much
a robot being fed by sugar, otherwise my battery would dwindle and
die. This robot got jammed and broke down. Its hardware could not
handle the software. Through Thetahealing, I removed many 'shoulds'
and 'musts' from the software. When I changed my diet, I gave the robot
a different kind of power supply. The robot had a discontinued power
supply: at times, it gave peak performance and other times the battery
would overheat, lowering its performance.

I reconnected with my life force while in Greece at the Osho Afroz
Meditation Center. I would do at least two active meditations a day. Unlike
still meditations, those involved movement and shaking. While there, I was
introduced to conscious dancing: a form of individual barefoot dancing
with no learnt steps. The instructions are simple: connect to the music,
find your flow and express yourself. At first, I struggled to find any kind of

flow. I felt like a dead woman. I would feel nauseous, tears would stream down my face, and I would scream. So much energy was trapped in this body and had created stiffness and pain. As my body softened, I was able to express myself and release some of my emotions. I began experiencing moments of aliveness that connected to the fire in me, my life force. I could not sustain this fire though: it would easily burn out.

After I left Greece, and for months afterwards, I spent thirty minutes each day dancing. I was determined to do all that I possibly could to call my energy back. My energy kept rising and crashing very much like an unreliable power supply. Then one day, as I was watching the "Heal documentary", Dr. Kelly Turner caught my attention. She mentioned nine things cancer patients do to achieve radical remission:

1. Radically changing your diet
2. Taking control of your health
3. Following your intuition
4. Using herbs and supplements
5. Releasing suppressed emotions
6. Embracing social support
7. Deepening your spiritual connection
8. Having strong reasons for living

I was astonished at how those eight points summarized what I had been doing so far, with the exception of the herbs and supplements. While I was not a cancer patient, I had done them in no particular order in an effort to feel alive again. That gave me some comfort. *I was heading in the right direction.* Yet, my energy was still lagging. The pain in my body reminded me of my maternal grandmother in her old age. We could not touch her. She felt pain everywhere. I did not want to end up like her, and I was determined to get in touch with this pain so that I could release it. I was not ready to give up and wanted to regain the energy necessary to achieve any dream I wished.

My friend Pravas, whom I had met in India highly recommended Biodynamic Breathwork and Trauma Release System (BBTRS). I had done some breathwork towards the end of my stay in Greece, and then participated in a breath festival in Turkey. It connected me with a boiling inner volcano that, at that time, was too much for me to handle. After my downtime in Lebanon, I now felt ready to enter this active boiler and lower its temperature to a level that was tolerable to me. Pravas had mentioned that the founder of BBTRS, Giten Tonkov and his partner Nisarga Dobosz, were offering a certification path. I contacted them and enrolled in their upcoming course in Poland. I spent a month in Poland attending three courses in Qigong, healing development trauma and BBTRS. We stayed in the countryside. It was spring time: the birds were in a constant symphony and nature was coming alive again, just like me. The setting was nurturing for this kind of deep work.

My motivation to do a whole week of qigong was engrained in a desire to learn a sequence of movement to cultivate positive energy. The Master, Simon Calder, is the embodiment of a loving presence. He was quick to manage my expectation: "Qigong is not about memorizing and repeating a sequence of movements, but rather how you move." Over a week, we slowly moved and stretched our myo-fascial tissue to purge the body from toxic energy. The myo-fascial tissue is the connective gelatin-like tissue that wraps our structure of bones, muscles and nerves together, very much like a sac. When it's flexible, our body is able to move with less effort. I had an AHA moment: *movement is not about more but rather less: how to move with less effort.* I practiced slowness through moving slower, then moved on to my slowest.

Since I happened to be in Poland, and had a free week until the breathwork workshop, I signed up to take a Healing Developmental Trauma course. I came to understand the disconnection between my body and mind. Given the war circumstances surrounding my birth, I cut the life force from my body in order not to feel the pain, as an unconscious survival mechanism. Instead, I lived in my mind, becoming a sharp intellectual. It's no wonder why I kept experiencing such an interruption in my energy flow towards my body. I also came to understand that my body was in 'freeze mode', very much like a gazelle when attacked by a lion. I freeze when I am overwhelmed, Even more, I become lethargic and sleep a lot. Whenever distressed, my energy and emotions shut down while my mind becomes vibrant, alive with possibilities that may or may not be negative.

In his book The Body Keeps the Score: Brain, Mind, and Body in

<u>Healing Trauma</u>, Bessel A. van der Kolk talks about how our bodies are a reflection of our traumas. He explains:

> Trauma victims cannot recover until they become familiar with and befriend the sensations in their bodies. Being frightened means that you live in a body that is always on guard. Angry people live in angry bodies. The bodies of child-abuse victims are tense and defensive until they find a way to relax and feel safe. In order to change, people need to become aware of their sensations and the way that their bodies interact with the world around them. Physical self-awareness is the first step in releasing the tyranny of the past.

Body awareness became my new frontier. While I had been treating my body with loving kindness for about two years, we were somehow still disconnected. I did not trust it, and I would often feel betrayed by my lack of energy and pain. Thanks to Biodynamic Breath and Trauma Release, I developed greater inner awareness. I would close my eyes and feel my heartbeat. *Is it fast or slow? I would feel my lungs expanding and contracting as they breathed in the air of life for me. How easy is the breathing? I would walk a bit and check my balance. Am I grounded or not? Is my walk heavy or light? Where am I feeling the lightness or heaviness in my body? What is the sensation like? Is it a block weighing my body down? Or rather itchiness or a burn?*

Rather than taking clues from the outside, I became more attentive to my inner voice, body signals, and allowed them to guide my decision-making in the present moment. If I am heading straight, and my body is asking me to go in the opposite direction, I now listen and change course. When I find myself restless in a gathering that I had been eagerly looking forward to, I give myself permission to leave. I am now more aware of what sensations kick in with each and every person I interact with. Sensations are not controlled by the mind. They fluctuate and respond to an unpredictable smell, movement, sound or view.

As I began to breathe deeper, I encountered unpleasant body sensations. I came to discover that as children, we unconsciously develop a shallow breath in order not to feel painful sensations. I began to befriend this unease. I did not need to run away. I felt the sensations and breathed through them. At times, I cried, other times I laughed, or sang. I avoided any mind games, and, instead, stayed in the course following the sensation to its root. When we breathe through the discomfort, contracted muscles eventually relax. I did not die, rather I was alive, and feeling more so with every breath I took.

Thanks to breathwork, I am one with my body, able to connect to any sensation in the present moment. My body feels like home. I am safe in this vessel. Whenever I catch myself fighting with my shadows, I know it's time for an intervention and an adjustment. Through meditation, I am able to connect to my state of being and devise what is exactly needed for an improvement. Vocal cords exercises awaken the energy inside and clear away any blockages I may be experiencing. Dancing shakes my energy up, releasing unneeded tensions, and bringing my life force back. Qigong slows my body and makes me more fluid, bringing an overall sensation of vitality. Yoga pauses stretch the latent pain in my muscle, taking away my stiffness by improving flexibility. Self-massage awakens my body.

As I learn to live in my body, I am feeling an increased life force. I am alive when I dance. I am alive when I write. I am alive when I sing. I am alive in the company of loved ones. I am alive when I cook and clean the house. I am alive when I am at peace with my body and flowing in its rhythm. Nature makes me alive. Giving a healing session makes me alive. When I am alive, I am absorbed in the moment. I am effortlessly in flow, thanks to an endless supply of energy. My emotions are alive. My body is alive. My heart is alive.

There are moments when my batteries are drained for no obvious reason. I ask myself: is there something that has recently pissed me off? I still have a high tolerance level for people's negativity, and I hate being pushy. I am more aware that when I unconsciously repress my anger, I am redirecting my life force to keep the anger locked in. I have now given myself an invitation to be angry: *yes I am allowed to be angry. It's ok to be angry. I know how to be angry. I know when to be angry.* Being angry is healthy and acceptable, not shameful, embarrassing, or hurtful, rather it is a relief to be able to express oneself.

There are days when fear kicks in, and I feel like hiding under the bed covers. I allow that consciously. After I calm down, I imagine myself being protected by the light of the sun. Other times, I anchor myself in my power, and imagine myself taking back all the powers that I have surrendered to others. There are times when I just embrace my frozenness and enjoy the intellectual pursuits that keep me hanging in there, alive and well. No need to force anything. After all, I have forced myself into many situations in the past. For now, I practice loving kindness.

As a morning person, I am energized from sunrise to sunset and useless at night. I used to giggle at my paternal grandmother who would go to bed at five or six p.m. during winter and wake up before dawn. My dad would sleep a bit later around eight or nine p.m. and wake up by sunrise. While growing up, my cousins would play tricks on me to test what would get me out of bed. That was extremely annoying! As I became older, no amount of food nor drink gave me enough energy to enjoy night outings and socialization. I now realize that, to me, being awake at night is self-torture. I now accept my nature and listen to my body. I embrace my sleep early genes without shame and don't attempt to change my body clock.

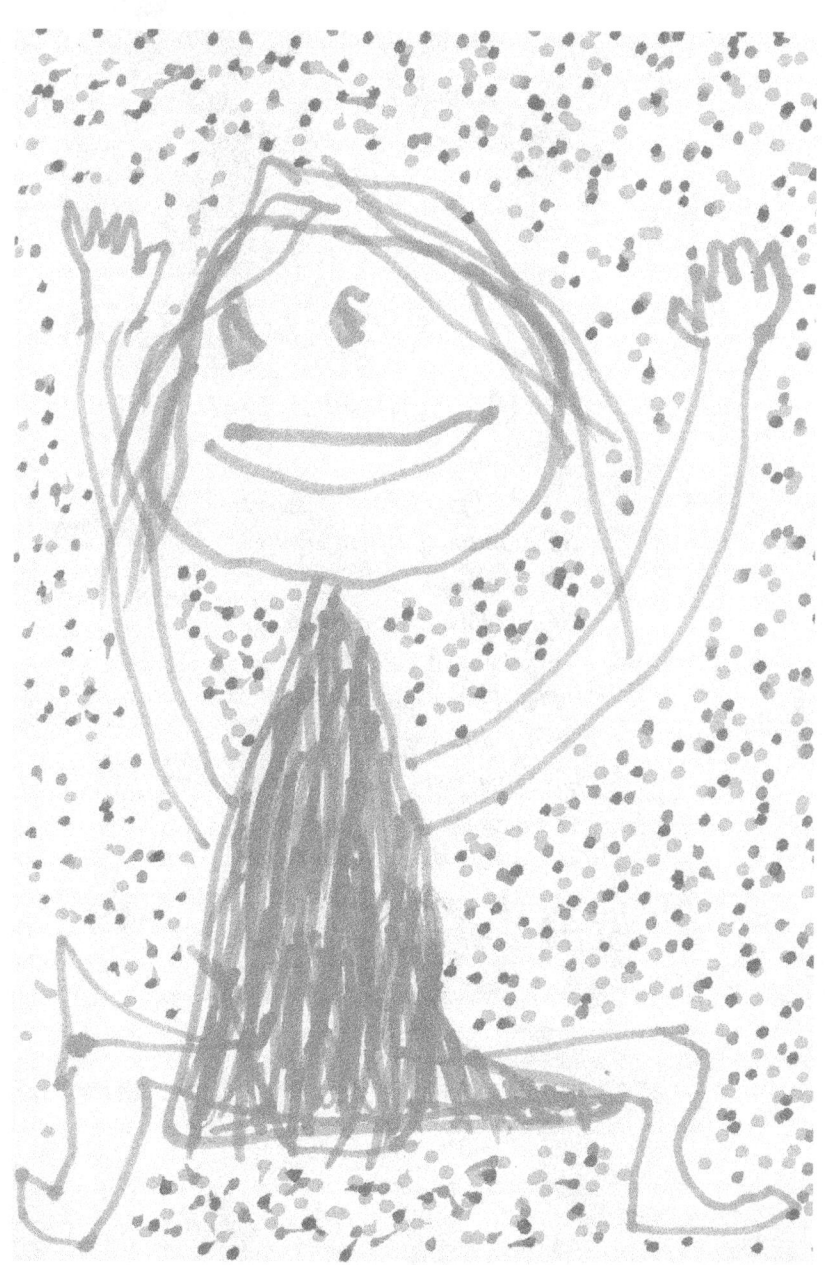

The joy of aliveness

■

ABUNDANCE

I possess love
Surrounding me from above!
I possess gratitude,
Giving me a soft attitude.
I possess kindness,
That I share with fondness.
I possess grace
Spreading in my body and face.
I possess joy and tranquility
Growing all the way to infinity.
I possess abundance,
Oh God, thank you for this allowance.

■

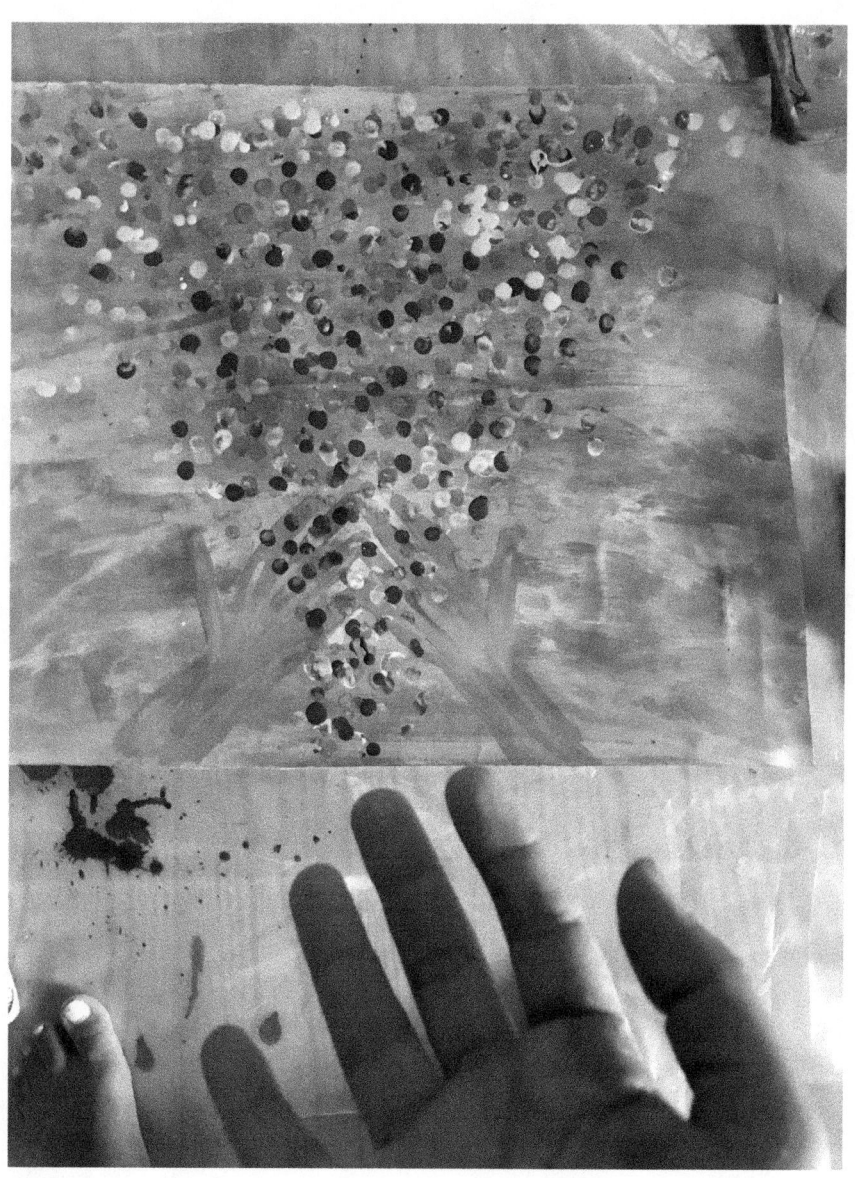

A burst of creativity

CHAPTER 15

EMBRACING LIFE

■

Just let go of how your life should be and embrace the life that is trying to work its way into your consciousness.
- Caroline Myss

Growing up, I aspired to be a superwoman. Climbing the corporate ladder was my reason for living. Following the bicycle accident, I gradually let go of an ordered life in favor of uncertainty and disorganization. After fourteen months of travel, I settled in Lebanon. I came from Poland with renewed energy and inspiration to begin my healing practice. I was ready to give back and allow others to experience what had helped me.

My school friend Zeina had been pushing me to start my healing practice for months. I had so far enjoyed caring for friends and family on the go, yet feared the constraints of a new structure that might be binding to my energy again. As I struggled with the idea of asking for money, the universe sent me my first paying customer. She needed help and gave me the courage to start. I became a healer and food addiction counselor, supporting others to lead happier and healthier lives. I began offering sessions in biodynamic breathwork and trauma release, Thetahealing, and food addiction recovery. Thanks to my diversified know-how, I was able to support clients with stress release and relaxation, building on my knowledge of Osho therapies, meditation, Reiki, Qigong and Thai yoga massage. I was able to offer a personalized approach to support the needs of each person, using my intuition and the insights I have gained from my personal transformation.

Fulfillment is not about being happy all the time. As I embarked on my journey, I thought that being slim would make me happy. Then, I thought quitting my career and becoming free would make me happy. I later thought having a significant other would make me happy. What I have found is that happiness is not a milestone. Inner peace is an ability to feel the high and the low, and be able to navigate through them. I now live in playful flow with the present moment. I embrace life and allow its wind to direct me. There are days when I don't feel good, and that's Ok. I allow myself to just be, in whatever state of being I happen to be. I embrace the turbulence knowing that the storm shall pass. Sometimes, I am at peace with myself and other times I am at war, and that is Ok. I now enjoy the little pleasures of life, those physical sensations that come when my body feels good. Ironically, my body never felt good before.

I am now blessed with a new home. I am grateful for this eighteen-month transition during which I made an inner and outer pilgrimage traveling to the US, Greece, Ghana, UAE, India and Poland. In between those travels, I bonded with my parents, whom I had left when I was eighteen. As I settled into my new home, I felt I had completed a full circle and was now back to my base, reunited with my furniture, carpets, wall decorations and other objects that I had acquired and formed an attachment to along the course of my life. Somehow, this marked the beginning of the next half of my life.

To make things more interesting, turbulence began in Lebanon again. A revolution started as a result of popular discontent with the political class' corruption. A banking, economic, and political crisis ensued. People stayed on the streets for months interrupting the daily flow of life. The government is bankrupt and is holding people's money in banks hostage. This is a long-term crisis with no quick fix. Each person is going through a change curve. Politicians and bankers are mourning a past that no longer exists. The people are angry about their stolen money. We are all struggling to adjust to the crash of the Lebanese economy and state. The Covid 19 pandemic began amidst Lebanon's meltdown. Somehow, after all this fury, a time of forced isolation grounded everyone at home and made life further uncertain.

I am open to the mystery that is life. Every day, I practice playfulness with the uncertainty, and trust that some blessings will emerge. Starting a new life in times of crisis might not be the easiest thing. However, I trust that there is a certain universal wisdom for this restructuring. Perhaps, God made me return to Lebanon to be of service to others during this turn of events. I just allow life to lead me. Rumi wisely said: *"As you begin to walk on the way, the way appears."* I do not worry much about what will happen tomorrow or the day after. I focus on the right now. The present moment is all that counts. Yesterday is gone and tomorrow is unborn. I do not make grand plans as I have stopped living with futuristic plans that impose a fast pace that is detrimental to my health. For today, I tend to my wellbeing. When I am well, all will flow allowing the universe to connect me with whomever needs me. Just as Imam Shafii said: *"My heart is at ease knowing that what was meant for me will never miss me, and that what misses me was never meant for me."*

Allowing life to
support and
shape me

$$\neq$$

forcing to fit
in existing
life

I am happy
I am home
I love myself
YES YES
HOURRAY
WAWGOOO
YE YYYYY

■

EASE

I visualize ease,
And feel its lightness in my knees.
Ease is settling here,
Its grace is the new norm,
Coming in every sweet form.
Ease is the flow
Allowing my life to glow.

■

CHAPTER 16

HEALING THE HUNGER

■

We don't know what we need, and as long as we stay in
the hungry ghost mode, we'll never know.

- Gabor Mate

Three years ago, I embarked on a path of physical, emotional and spiritual transformation. Over my journey, I have come to realize that I was born with a hole. The emptiness has always been with me. My mom was a disciplinarian who believed in feeding schedules. As a baby, I developed an anxious relationship with food as my hunger would be ignored. I know the hungry ghost very well. It has accompanied me all of my life.

Whenever the hungry ghost acts out, I initiate an inner dialogue with myself: *Do I really need to eat right now? How true is my hunger? Isn't my brain sending a false message?* Food is not the solution in those situations because the last time I acted on a food urge, my problem was not solved. When I am unable to calm my unease, I distract myself by walking around, or doing something physical that involves moving the body such as cooking, running errands, sorting things, or connecting with loved ones.

The hungry ghost arises when anger and fear are masked. They usually manifest in a tense gut asking to be filled. *What is my hungry ghost trying to tell me? What unease am I suppressing? Am I revolting against my needs not being met? Do I know what those needs are? Am I afraid and looking for safety? Am I disoriented and seeking direction? Am I vulnerable and desiring tender love and care? Am I rebelling? Am I affirming my right to existence? Am I expressing my appetite for life? Am I bored? Am I ignoring something that is pissing me off?* My feeling of hunger is an invitation to enter my innerness and meet the need that is seeking my attention. I may not have the answers immediately. I journal every day and reflect about what my body is trying to tell me. Through journaling, valuable insights surface into my consciousness and anchor me in the goodness that is my life.

When the hungry ghost is activated, I welcome it as a danger sign that my mind, body and soul are disconnected. I recognize that keeping those three in balance is the foundation for sustaining the weight-loss. My hungry ghost is an invitation to slow down and reach within. I cancel plans and rearrange priorities to mobilize all my resources inwards. I switch to an inner nurse tending to my fragile self. This process usually involves several days of self-care to bring back my whole being back into balance.

My journey of recovery from food addiction continues. I follow a food plan consisting of four measured meals a day free from sugar, flour, and I fast in between my meals. I have a network of fellow recovering food addicts. We regularly video call to discuss our challenges of the moment, and offer each other advice.

My commitment to my plan comes from the certainty I have towards my aliveness, especially in these times of deep uncertainty. Today, I know I have a choice: do I fill my unease and emptiness with physical food or do I seek the less tangible? I enjoy the mystery that is my body, a mystery that is in constant evolution. I commit to being a loving presence in this glorious vessel. When I am in contact with my deepest needs, I know I will not resort to overeating. After all, change and growth are seldom a straight line. You progress as you go, venturing into new paths through peaks, valleys and detours. While there is a beginning in any journey, there is no end as long as we are alive.

I am angry
Wasssssss
I want to eat
can you hear me?
I am angry
I am here
I am angry
can you hear me?

I am hungry for love
hungry to be loved
hungry to be hugged
hungry to be touched
hungry to be one ONE
hungry to unite
hungry to melt

food is not Love
food is food
food is nourish
overeating is poisonous

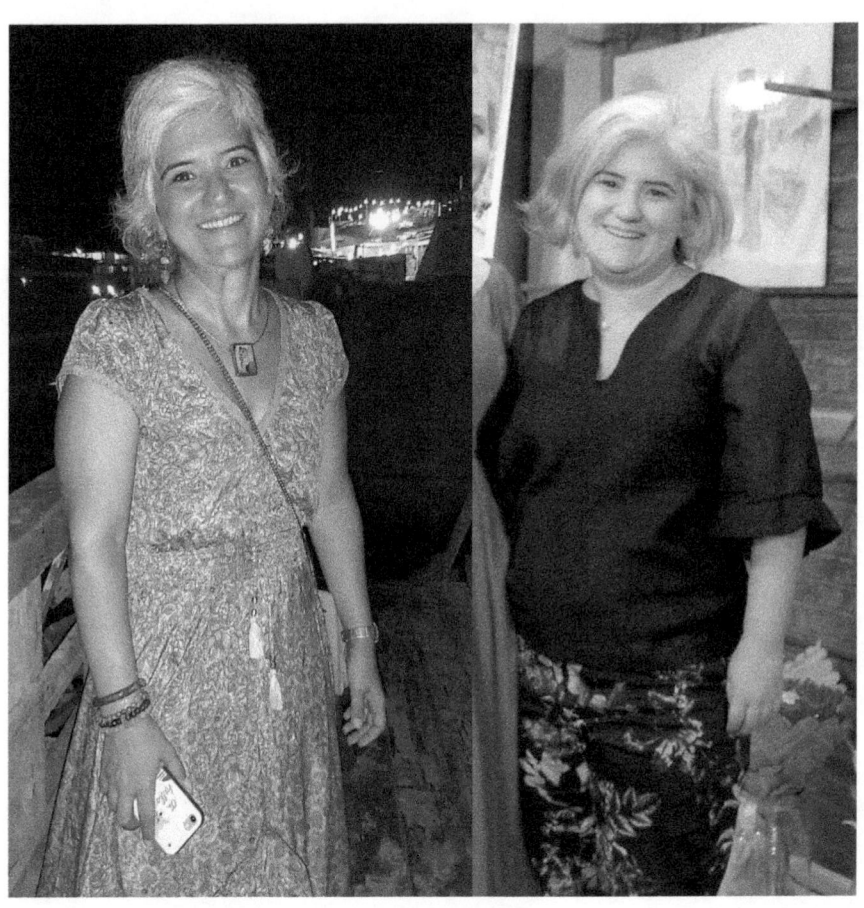

A journey of three years

BIBLIOGRAPHY

Aron, Elaine N. *The Highly Sensitive Person*. Harmony Books, 2016

Bonheim, Jalaja. *Aphrodite's Daughters: Women's Sexual Stories and the Journey of the Soul*. Fireside, 1997

Bradshaw, John. *Healing the Shame that Binds You*. Health Communications, 2005

Bradshaw, John. *Homecoming*. Piatkus, 1999

Brown, Jeff. *An Uncommon Bond*. Enrealment Press, 2015

Foster, Jeff. *The Joy of True Meditation*. New Sarum Press, 2019

Hay, Louise. *You Can Heal Your Life*. Hay House, 2005

Levine, Amir and Heller, Rachel. *Attached: The New Science of Adult Attachmenet and How It Can Help You Find and Keep Love*. Tarcher Perigee, 2011

Mate, Gabor. *In the Realm of the Hungry Ghosts: Close Encounters with Addiction*. North Atlantic Books, 2010

Osho. *God Is Dead: Now Zen Is the Only Living Truth*. Osho Media International, 1997

Osho. *The Fish in The Sea is Not Thirsty*. Wisdom Tree, 2008

Pierce Thompson, Susan. *Bright Line Eating*. Hay House, 2017

Premartha & Svarup. *Twice Born: Healing the Past Creating a New Future.* Book on Demand

Tarman, Vera with Werdell, Phil. *Food Junkies.* Dundurn, 2014

Tolle, Eckhart. *A New Earth: Awakening to your Life's Purpose.* Penguin Books, 2016

Tonkov, Giten. *Feel to Heal: Releasing Trauma Through Body Awareness and Breathwork Practice.* Biodynamic Breathwork and Trauma Release Institute, 2019

Turner, Kelly. *Radical Remission: Surviving Cancer Against All Odds.* Harper One, 2014

Van Der Kolk, Bessel. *The Body Keeps the Score: Brain, Mind and the Body in the Healing of Trauma.* Penguin Books, 2014

Werdell Phil and Roccio Beth, *Treating Food Addiction: Book 1: The basics.* Evergreen Publishing, 2017

Werdell, Phil and Foushi, Mary. *Food Plans for Food Addiction Recovery: a Physical and Spiritual Tool.* Evergreen Publishing, 2015

ABOUT THE AUTHOR

Rouba Chalabi, after years of struggling with overeating, found herself on a path of radical physical, emotional and spiritual transformation - resulting, finally, in a weight-loss she could healthfully sustain. Inspired to become a healer and food addiction counselor, she left a twenty-year career in public policy and communication to return to her native Lebanon. Through her private practice there, Rouba now helps people overcome similar struggles to discover their authentic selves.

She can be reached at
E-mail: rouba.chalabi@icloud.com
Facebook: Rouba Chalabi
Instagram: roubachalabi and abstinent.salads
Twitter: @rouba_chalabi
Linked In: Rouba Chalabi